# Pregnancy: Put Yourself in Her Shoes

*A Complete Guide for Future Fathers to Understand and Support Their Pregnant Partners*

By MK DAVIS

### About the Author:

### MK DAVIS

*MK is a pleased married man, passioned by his family. Father of three (two girls and one boy), he has always been keen to be fully involved in fatherhood. Because of his natural empathy, he also always wanted to share full experience of both sides of being a parent with his wife: the joy but also the burden of pregnancy. The best way to do so: "put yourself in her shoes".*

*Being trained in feminine psychology and biology, MK shares his experiences and knowledge in this book, as a guide for future fathers to understand and support their pregnant partners.*

*According to his own wife: this is the best piece of advice any future moms can share with their partners for him to be a "perfect pregnancy supporter" and an excellent future dad!*

*Dedicated to my lovely wife and my lovely mother for their help and constant support...*

# Table of contents

## Chapter 3: Surviving the First Trimester

# Introduction

Congratulations on trusting *"Pregnancy: Put Yourself in Her Shoes,"* and thank you for doing so. Just by purchasing this book, you have shown that you are interested in being a superstar dad and partner who is engaged, informed, and as supportive as possible throughout pregnancy and the life of your child. You should congratulate yourself just for taking this initiative!

The following chapters will discuss everything that you need to know about pregnancy, so you can support your partner in every way that counts. You'll receive education on what she is experiencing – from physical symptoms to confusing emotions. You'll learn how the baby develops in the three trimesters of pregnancy and how you can help ease any uncomfortable side effects your partner feels. You'll also find out how to take an active role in preparing your home and mindset for fatherhood. On top of all this, you'll learn how to be an active, supportive, and helpful advocate for your partner during the entire painful process of labor and delivery.

Although there is no substitute for the experience of pregnancy, labor, and delivery, this book will prepare you in every way possible to be sympathetic to your partner's needs throughout the nine months and beyond. Read through this book and then use it as a reference whenever you come across questions or unknown situations and don't know how to support your partner.

There are plenty of books on this subject on the market, so thanks again for choosing this one! Every effort was made to ensure it is full of as much useful information as possible. Please enjoy!

# Chapter 1: Before She's Even Pregnant

For some husbands, partners, and fathers-to-be, it may be a little too late to read this chapter. That's okay! No matter when you have decided to educate yourself and become the most supportive partner possible, your efforts should be applauded.

Some of you have realized that conceiving a child does not come easily to everyone. Conception can be a very lengthy, difficult, emotionally taxing, and financially draining process for some couples. This chapter provides information and helpful hints so that you can be as educated and supportive to your partner as possible during these pre-pregnancy days, weeks, months, or even years. The process may be emotionally draining for you as well. Make sure you reach out for any help and support you may need so that you can be there for her.

## Conceiving Naturally

Of course, in an ideal world, just deciding to "start trying" would result in an instant pregnancy. But nature doesn't always make it that easy. There are plenty of barriers between and her egg; in fact, it's a miracle any of us were born at all!

Of the millions of sperm, a man ejaculates during sex, only about 100,000 make it past his partner's cervix at the entrance to the uterus. These sperms have managed to run the gauntlet of acidic vaginal secretions. Of these 100,000 sperms, only a measly 200 make it into one of the two fallopian tubes, where a ready-to-be fertilized egg is waiting – that is if your timing is right and your partner is ovulating (producing an egg). Fortunately, there is much sperm to start with because such a small percentage of them survive the journey. In the end, it's a race to see which one of your sperm emerges as the champion and fertilizes the egg by breaking into it.

After the egg has been fertilized, it moves down the fallopian tube and into the uterus or womb. It begins dividing into multiple cells, and soon the tiny cluster of cells begins implanting in the lining of the uterus wall, which is also known as the endometrium. This little cluster of cells then starts the process of transforming into an embryo. After eight weeks of pregnancy, the embryo is called a fetus. At this point, you and your partner may be aware that your baby is on the way.

# What You Can Do to Increase the Odds

Like many sports victories, getting pregnant is a matter of having quality equipment and right timing. If you follow these helpful hints, you will increase your chances of getting pregnant:

## Get in shape

Just like prospective mothers, you can improve the odds of conception by being as healthy as possible. Now is an ideal time to quit smoking, take it easy on alcohol, stop doing any recreational drugs, start exercising, and eat healthily. You should probably be following this advice anyway.

## Let gravity help

Try to keep your partner lying down – propping her hips up with a pillow to help gravity even more – rather than getting up and heading to the bathroom right after sex. You'll help those precious sperm get to their destination by keeping your partner horizontal with her pelvis tilted upward. So, cuddle up or do whatever it takes to keep her in bed! Remember – every little bit helps!

## Watch the calendar

Ovulation is when an egg is produced and ready for fertilization. It occurs on approximately day

14 of a 28-day menstrual cycle, with day one being the first day of your partner's period. So, plan for that time to be your "business time." If your partner's cycle is irregular or you need more reassurance, try an ovulation test kit to see whether the time is right for romance. Ovulation test kits – sold over the counter at pharmacies and large chain stores – are urine tests that detect hormones, much like pregnancy test kits. Look for them near the pregnancy test kits in the family planning section.

## Get a health check

Your partner will have to go through all manner of doctor visits during her pregnancy, but you are not entirely off the hook. To make sure your sperm is in the best shape possible, a physical exam for you is a good idea. Your doctor can check for any signs of sexually transmitted disease, any anatomical problems such as an undescended testicle, and any other issues of which you may not be aware.

## Check the safety of any medication you are taking

Prescribed medication and over-the-counter drugs can have an adverse effect on you as well as mom or baby, so check with your doctor before taking anything during the baby-making process – and beyond.

## Practice!

Have sex at least once a day when your partner is ovulating. If you feel a little put off by scheduled intimate time, have sex at least every other day – even when she's not ovulating. You never know what might happen. Being "in the mood" for sex has also been shown to help you conceive. Do some research on positions that aid conception and try them out, too!

## Don't stress

Research has shown that stress can affect your partner's ovulation, so try not to get too worked up about not getting pregnant right away. Good things take time and worrying about it won't make things happen any faster. Wanting to get pregnant is an excellent excuse for having lots of sex, so enjoy it for a while. If your partner is age 35 or younger, the average time until conception after you begin trying is six months. Yes, that seems like an eternity when making a baby is foremost in your minds. But try to relax and help your partner to do the same. Give her back rubs, encourage her to book some time at a spa, and take part in doing the housework, too. The less stressed she is, the better her chances of getting pregnant.

# When It's Just Not Happening

You've been trying for months. And trying. And trying. But conception is just not happening. You feel like you're getting sick of sex, which is a problem you thought you would *never* encounter. But you may be feeling that sex is the last thing you'd like to do. Guess what? Being sex-tired is a normal feeling for men after trying to conceive for months upon months. So, don't beat yourself up. Besides, your partner is probably experiencing the same feelings at this point.

Couples under 35 years of age who have been having regular unprotected sex for a year and haven't become pregnant are considered to be infertile. Those over 35 years old are called sterile after six months of trying without conception. If either of these cases describes you, it may be time to talk to your doctor about getting some help.

It's not time to panic yet, and you need to do the best you can to reassure your partner if you're having trouble conceiving. Tell her that you are there for her. Remind her that there are still plenty of things that you can do and that the two of you don't have all the information yet. Assuming a worst-case scenario will only cause unnecessary stress for her.

# Understanding What Can Go Wrong

Approximately one in six couples have an issue with getting pregnant. There are a lot of factors in both partners that can cause infertility, but let's look at what factors could be affecting you for the moment. Problems on the male front – meaning that your boys don't swim as well as they should – can account for 40 percent of "infertile" couples not being able to get pregnant. Low sperm counts, blockages to sperm ejaculation, poor sperm motility (which means the direction they move – going around in circles doesn't help make a baby), and sperm with an abnormal shape account for most fertility problems among men.

The following factors can contribute to infertility in men:

- **Anatomical problems** such as erectile dysfunction or blockage caused by a varicose vein called a varicocele that connects to the testicle.

- **Regular exposure to harmful substances** such as heavy metals in your environment.

- **Lifestyle**, such as smoking or taking drugs, can slow sperm.

- **Overheated sperm** caused by taking frequent hot baths or wearing tight-fitting underwear or pants (even jeans can be a problem if they're too tight).

- **Sexually transmitted diseases**, such as gonorrhea or chlamydia.

In 40 percent of cases of male infertility, the cause may not be known. Either way, going for a checkup is a good idea. So, now it's time to be a man and own up to this task – if there's a problem, at least you'll know, and the chances are that you can do something about it. This knowledge will reduce stress overall, and your partner will love and appreciate you even more for having a checkup.

If the issue is *not* with you, but your partner, try to be aware that this can be an extremely rough time for her for her. She may be feeling like a bit of a failure. A lot of women believe that being able to carry and nurture a child is an essential part of being a woman, and not being able to do this may leave her feeling inadequate. As her partner, you're in the best position to help her feel just as whole as a woman no matter what.

# Exploring Other Options

If you and your partner are having trouble conceiving a child, the first step is to talk to your doctor. In some cases, lifestyle factors may be holding you back, and if the problem is a blockage, surgery could help. But in other cases, it may be time to consider assisted reproductive technologies and working with a fertility specialist.

The following are some of the treatments you may want to talk about with your doctor:

## Intrauterine insemination (IUI)

Your semen is collected, given a bit of a cleanup, then inserted into your partner's vagina, uterus, or fallopian tubes. For the semen collection process, there may be a plastic cup and some dirty magazines involved – but hey, it's all for a good cause! This treatment is available for sperm with low motility, meaning they can't get to the egg without help. It may also assist in the case of other fertility issues.

## In vitro fertilization (IVF)

This process is also known as making a "test tube" baby. Your partner is given hormone treatments to kick-start her ovulation and cause her to release multiple fertile eggs at once. When she is ovulating, she goes through a procedure in which the eggs are harvested. The doctor mixes the collected eggs with your sperm and given a chance to be fertilized. The fertilized eggs are then put into your partner's uterus. Then you wait to see whether they implant into the uterine wall.

## Intracytoplasmic sperm injection (ICSI)

Rather than mix sperm and egg and wait to see which eggs are fertilized, sperm is injected straight into the egg. As with IVF, the fertilized eggs are placed into your partner's uterus, where hopefully one plants.

If you do use IVF or other assisted reproductive technology, you should know a few things. For one thing, there is an increased chance of multiple births. According to recent research, on average one in four IVF treatments results in multiple pregnancies compared with one in 80 naturally conceived pregnancies.

With IVF, sometimes two embryos are placed into the uterus, increasing the chances of having twins. If your partner is under age 35 and has no uterine abnormalities, some clinics will limit you to putting back no more than two embryos at a time. This is because the chance of complications during pregnancy and birth is higher with multiple pregnancies than with a single baby.

Another good thing to know is that medical intervention is often highly successful for couples who are having trouble conceiving naturally. About two-thirds of couples dealing with infertility do have a baby through assisted reproductive technology, so it is worth finding out about these options. Ask your doctor all your questions, even if they seem embarrassing.

# What If Nothing is Working?

For some couples, even assisted reproductive technology does not result in successful conception. The realization that you are unlikely to have a biological child of your own can be devastating for a couple. Although you should remain hopeful throughout the process and keep an upbeat attitude for the sake of your emotional health and supporting your partner, you should also mentally prepare yourself for the worst. Sometimes, even after multiple rounds of IVF, a couple still cannot successfully conceive.

You and your partner should maintain open and honest communication throughout this process. Check in with her regularly, to see how she's holding up, emotionally and physically. Sometimes the process of trying to conceive is so psychologically and financially draining that it can drive a wedge between partners. You should try to avoid that situation at all costs! Keep the lines of communication open, so you know when you have hit your stopping point. In the end, it may be a relief to decide to stop trying and explore other options. Also, don't be afraid to suggest psychological counseling for the two of you to help you get through the grief you may be experiencing as a result of the difficulty in conceiving a child. Additionally, support groups may be available for couples who have shared similar experiences.

## Considering Adoption

While this guide is not meant to be an adoption handbook, it is worth mentioning briefly. Some couples consider this option after IVF has failed, and some think about it without even trying any medical intervention to help with conception. Being unable to conceive a child does not mean that you cannot be parents.

Adopting a child means that you take on parental rights and responsibilities of looking after that child as you would if you were his biological parents. That is a lifetime of responsibility. It can be easy to love your child unconditionally, and you have to decide whether you're willing and able to do that for a child who is not biologically yours.

Many adoptions these days are open adoptions, which means the child and his birth parents stay in touch with each other. Lawyers who specialize in adoption, private agencies, and the child welfare system are all potential sources to assist with adoption and matching parents with a child.

The number of babies who are put up for adoption in the United States and other first-world countries is much lower now than it was a generation ago. Some couples look into adopting a child from overseas. Americans adopt more children from China than from any other country, but many children are also adopted from Eastern European nations such as Ukraine, as well as from countries such as Haiti.

Whether you go the home-grown route or travel overseas, the adoption process is a lengthy and often expensive one. There are police and background checks, information evenings to attend, and visits to your home from social workers. Once you have jumped through all the official hoops, your profile may be put into a pool waiting to be selected by birth parents. This can take up to a year or more.

Just like trying to conceive a child, the adoption process can take an emotional toll on you and your partner. Again, it is critical to keep the communication lines open and share how you are feeling. Counseling and support groups may be beneficial to the two of you to get through the process with optimal communication and support as a couple.

# Chapter 2: Congratulations! Now What?

Once you have made it through conception to the point of your partner getting pregnant, whether it was a quick and easy process or a lengthy and difficult one, there are a whole host of new issues to face. But first – congratulations! You are now expecting a child. You and your partner are likely experiencing all kinds of emotions, including excitement, exhaustion, and anxiety.

This chapter educates you on things you need to consider at the very beginning of pregnancy and how you can support your partner through all the initial symptoms, emotions, and decisions.

## Possible Initial Pregnancy Symptoms

If you have been trying to conceive, you and your partner are probably on high alert and already well-versed in the possible symptoms for which you should be on the lookout. However, just in case you aren't sure, or this pregnancy snuck up on you faster than you expected, here are some things your partner may be experiencing before the pregnancy is confirmed – and some ways that you can help with these symptoms:

## Swollen, sore breasts

As quickly as two weeks into the pregnancy, her breasts may be feeling tender and painful as a result of hormonal changes. Or they may feel fuller and heavier. If they are sore, be sensitive and don't touch! You can enjoy the sight but keep your hands off, please.

## Exhaustion

At the beginning of the pregnancy, levels of the hormone progesterone are very high in your partner's body. This hormone causes her to feel very fatigued, so try to have some sympathy when she wants to nap in the middle of the day, or she's too tired to do anything. Low blood sugar levels and lowered blood pressure can also contribute to the overwhelming tiredness of early pregnancy. Be extra sensitive if she's feeling tired and know that she is not making it up. Just getting through a day at work may be more than your partner is up to at this point. You can help out with cooking meals and cleaning around the house and provide a quiet environment for her to nap.

## Slight bleeding or cramping

When the embryo implants in the wall of the uterus, your partner might experience abdominal cramps that feel like menstrual cramps. She may also have some slight bleeding, known as "spotting," that is a bit too early for an average period. The spotting and cramping can last from a few hours to a few days.

## Morning sickness

Nausea and vomiting can happen at any time of the day or night for a newly pregnant woman. Although this symptom may not start until several weeks into the pregnancy, for some it begins as early as the second week. This symptom is caused by rising levels of the hormone estrogen, along with an extremely heightened sense of smell. Be aware that your partner's nose may be extra sensitive and take care to help her avoid any odors that she finds repulsive.

Morning sickness does not pose a risk to the baby unless it's very severe, and it usually subsides after the first 12 weeks. It can come on anytime, but it is generally worse in the morning because your partner's stomach is empty. At its worst, morning sickness can be like having a hangover and being seasick at the same time, so no wonder your partner is off to the bathroom once again!

One thing that makes morning sickness worse is getting up on an empty stomach, so try having a plate of dry crackers or toast with a little jelly or peanut butter ready for your partner to nibble when she first wakes up. Other tips include eating smaller portions more often during the day, increasing intake of carbohydrates, and reducing consumption of fats. You might also try stimulating pressure points on the inner arms just above the wrists, which supposedly reduces nausea.

Morning sickness can get so severe that your partner may become dehydrated. The symptoms aren't always easy to spot, so double-check with your midwife, obstetrician, or primary care provider if your partner is having a rough time with morning sickness. He or she may prescribe medications to help reduce nausea. In severe cases, when your partner is unable to keep food or liquid down and is experiencing constant vomiting, you'll need to make a trip to the emergency room for intravenous fluids.

## Food cravings or aversions

Throughout pregnancy, your partner may turn up her nose at certain foods that she used to enjoy. She may also experience overwhelming cravings for other foods. This symptom may be particularly dramatic in the very early days of the pregnancy as a result of rapidly fluctuating hormones. You can help by avoiding the foods that make her feel sick, too. Sometimes the mere sight or smell of food can make her nauseous. You can also be at the ready to run out for any food she may be craving!

## Headaches

Because her blood circulation increases dramatically at the very beginning of pregnancy, she might experience frequent mild to moderate headaches. Whether you are sure she's pregnant or not, it's best to play it safe and avoid any over-the-counter nonsteroidal anti-inflammatories (NSAIDs) like ibuprofen. The painkiller acetaminophen (brand name Tylenol) is generally considered safe for pregnant women. Your partner may also be eternally grateful if you limit loud noises, help out with housework, and give her head and neck massages to help ease her headaches.

## Constipation

At the beginning of pregnancy, that pesky hormone progesterone can cause a slower passage of food through the intestines, leading to constipation. You can help by being sympathetic and encouraging your partner to ask her doctor about taking a stool softener and eating fiber-rich foods.

## Moodiness

Again, the hormones are to blame for this symptom. Your partner might be feeling especially emotional and teary, even when there is no apparent reason to feel sad. Tread lightly and never accuse her of being moody! Whether it's the hormones or not, treat all her emotions as entirely valid and provide a sympathetic shoulder to cry on whenever she needs it. Talk to your partner and figure out a way to communicate with her when she's in one of her moods because the hormones aren't going to go away any time soon.

## Faintness or dizziness

She may experience light-headedness or dizziness as her blood pressure drops, and blood vessels dilate. She may also experience faintness from low blood sugar. Be a hero by doing tedious household chores for her and always being ready to bring her a healthy snack.

## Higher body temperature

Sometimes women track their body temperature as a way of knowing when they are ovulating. Her temperature increases slightly right after she ovulates, and then remains at that level until her period begins. If her temperature stays at the slightly elevated level for more than two weeks, she might be pregnant. This symptom is not uncomfortable.

## Missing a period

This symptom is probably the most obvious and definitive of pregnancy symptoms. It is at this point when your partner can take an at-home pregnancy test and expect reasonably accurate results. She may have already experienced some of the other symptoms up to two weeks before the missed period so the time leading up to when she can take the test might seem interminable! You can be supportive by keeping her company and providing some relaxing, distracting, and time-consuming activities to help keep her mind off the agony of waiting.

# Testing for Confirmation

As soon as she missed a period or even displayed the slightest early pregnancy symptom, your partner probably raced off to the nearest pharmacy. Over-the-counter pregnancy tests can sometimes give inaccurate results, but they are more likely to give a false negative result than a false positive result. Testing the first-morning urine can improve accuracy because it is more concentrated at this time. Even if you have a positive result from an at-home test, the first thing you want to do is get confirmation from a doctor.

Make an appointment with a family doctor or obstetrician, who will test your partner's urine for the hormone human chorionic gonadotropin (HCG). HCG is the hormone responsible for the morning sickness and utter exhaustion your other half has to look forward to if she isn't already experiencing these symptoms. The doctor may also perform a gynecological exam on your partner to check the physical signs of pregnancy more closely. She may also have to go to the lab for a blood test to determine the exact level HCG in the blood. A blood test will help pinpoint how far along into the pregnancy she is.

Even your doctor can only provide a definitive answer when the pregnancy symptoms are apparent, which is around four weeks after fertilization. So, you should probably wait a little while before you start telling everyone the good news. You may want to wait awhile, until after the first ultrasound scan. We'll talk more about that in the next chapter. For now, keep this incredible news between the two of you.

Once you have confirmed the pregnancy, a celebration with your partner is in order! Treat her to a romantic evening at home or out on the town, depending on how she is feeling. Just remember that cigarettes, alcohol, and drugs are off the menu.

# Choosing a Prenatal Healthcare Provider

Before your partner progresses very far into the pregnancy, she'll need to have a confirmed prenatal healthcare provider, who will monitor her health and the health of the baby throughout the pregnancy and oversee the delivery of your baby. At one time, these appointments were strictly the domain of the pregnant woman and her doctor, but things have changed. You as the father can be much more involved now, which is a beautiful thing. Additionally, there are more choices about who you team up with for the journey to parenthood. Your partner's primary care doctor can refer her to pregnancy healthcare providers in your area.

The role of your prenatal care provider of choice is to guide you through the pregnancy, birth, and early weeks of your child's life. She monitors the baby's growth and well-being, and checks for conditions such as preeclampsia and gestational diabetes. She will also work with you to come up with a birth plan if your partner wants to create one, delivers your new baby, and helps you in the first few days after birth. This help may include getting your partner started with breastfeeding or helping with basic baby care tasks like bathing or changing a diaper. In general, your main maternity provider is your go-to if you have questions regarding health issues during the pregnancy. So, check with her before contacting other services or professionals.

It's true that a lot of attention at this time will be on the mom-to-be. But that doesn't mean that you cannot ask questions and have a say in the kind of care your partner and child receive. As the father, you have a critical role in the formation of your family. Do not feel embarrassed or afraid to ask about anything at all. Your partner will probably be impressed and appreciative of your initiative and willingness to participate in her care and the care of your unborn child.

It seems that there is a maze out there of midwives, birthing centers, obstetricians, and hospitals. Knowing who does what can help you and your partner decide where you would like your baby to be born and what kind of care she would like to receive during and immediately after birth:

## Family healthcare providers

Medical doctors, physician assistants, and nurse-practitioners may specialize in family medicine or general medical care, called internal medicine. They are not specialists in prenatal care or childbirth, but in rural settings, they may provide maternity care. Both nurse-practitioners who specialize in family medicine and physician assistants are often employed by and work with family medicine doctors.

## Certified nurse-midwives

These are trained health professionals who give prenatal care, deliver babies, help establish breastfeeding, and follow up for about four to six weeks after the birth to help when you are unsure about your baby's health. Lay midwives may have experience but no formal training. Midwives take a holistic approach to pregnancy and birth, and often counsel you as a family, acknowledging not just the physical challenges of becoming new parents, but also your mental and social well-being. They see pregnancy and birth as a natural process, not a medical one.

While they are trained in their field, they are not legitimate doctors and do not perform cesarean sections. If you choose to go with a midwife and complications arise during the pregnancy, she will most likely arrange for you to see an obstetrician. Certified nurse-midwives generally assist with hospital or birthing center births, while lay midwives or licensed midwives do home births. Lay midwives are not legally allowed to help with home births in many states. In some states, it's illegal to plan a home birth.

## Obstetricians

These are doctors who specialize in obstetrics, or the health of women and babies during pregnancy, birth, and after the birth, called the postpartum or postnatal period. They generally work in hospitals; few medical doctors in the United States participate in home births.

During the birth, midwives or hospital nurses are on hand throughout labor to monitor your partner and baby's progress. Obstetricians see their patients during labor as often as needed – more if your partner is high risk – and are present throughout the delivery itself. Obstetricians are primarily concerned with the physical health of the baby and mother, and generally don't assist with any nonmedical baby-care issues after birth, such as teaching you how to bathe your baby. However, hospital nurses can instruct you on anything that you have questions about before you discharge from the hospital. For help with general baby care after you leave the hospital, friends and family or an excellent prenatal class can be the most significant help. Lactation specialists offer excellent support for breastfeeding issues. Your doctor can recommend sources in your area.

You must talk with whoever you choose as your maternity healthcare provider about the options for where your baby can be born: at home, in a hospital, or a birthing center. The availability of options depends on where you live, the provider you have, and your partner's and baby's health and risk factors during the pregnancy.

Take the time to find the right maternity healthcare provider for your partner and you. Your family doctor may make a recommendation; family and friends may have suggestions based on their own experiences as well. Make sure you and your partner are satisfied and confident in your healthcare provider and that you have good chemistry. Things can get pretty hectic during pregnancy and birth, so you must make sure your partner is in good hands, and you're comfortable with your provider's personal and professional style. If you or your partner are ever not happy, consider making a change. Both of you should be 100 percent comfortable with your choice, but in reality, what's essential is that your partner is happy; she'll be seeing way more of her than you probably will.

## Things to Do to Celebrate and Start Preparing

In about nine months, your life will change forever. Now is the best time possible to do some of the things with your partner that may not be possible after your child is born. Here are a few things you might consider doing to celebrate your impending fatherhood, enjoy time with your partner, and prepare yourself:

- Enjoy lots of unprotected sex with your partner, since she's already pregnant. Keep in mind that she may be feeling too sick, exhausted, or overwhelmed for sex, so always be sensitive to her moods.
- Take a relaxing vacation with your partner. Vacationing will not be the same for the next 18 years or so, that's why you need to make the most of it now.
- Reflect on your own experience growing up and the things you want your child to experience.
- Sleep in late, cook brunch for you and your partner or go for picnics together.
- Splurge on a fancy restaurant dinner together or a day together at the spa.
- Start a journal, blog, or scrapbook to document the months leading up to your child's birth and make it a memento to give to your child when she's older. Your partner will be touched and pleased by this sentimental effort on your part!
- Research how to do massage, then practice on your partner. You can even purchase a few quality aromatherapy oils. She'll be very appreciative of your efforts throughout the next nine months!

- Take the time to touch bases with your partner regularly and discuss how you both are feeling. Ask how you can help. Be willing to *listen* to her thoughts, hopes, and fears, and resist the urge to "fix" anything unless she asks for help. She'll notice your efforts and be grateful since her emotions are probably all over the place right now.

# Chapter 3: Surviving the First Trimester

The easiest part of becoming a father is the whole pregnancy. You don't have to deal with any of the physical discomforts like morning sickness, leg cramps, or the inability to get out of bed without a crane. By the end of it, you may be tired of hearing about aches, pains, and cravings, but you must never act like you are tired of it. Trust and believe that she is far more tired of it all than you will ever be!

Just because you don't experience the physical symptoms doesn't mean that there is nothing for you to do during pregnancy. This is the time for you to step up and shine as a partner. Apart from all the preparations, there's all the stuff you can do with your partner to help her out and to get to know your developing child. Your partner needs a strong man for the end part, the birth of your baby.

Pregnancy consists of three trimesters, and each one has its ups and downs. Although there is generally a little debate about exactly when each trimester begins and ends, you can take a mathematical approach to it. Since pregnancy is 40 weeks long (with the first day of "pregnancy" being the first day of her last period), you might say the first trimester is 13 and 1/3 weeks long.

Some people round up or down and say it is 13 or 14 weeks long. In this chapter, you'll learn what to expect during the first trimester, the symptoms and emotions your partner may be experiencing, and how you can best support her during this time.

## Deciding When (and How) to Tell People

Every couple has different ideas of when the best time to tell their loved ones the great news might be, and how they want to make the blessed announcement. Some couples prefer to wait until they are safely out of the first trimester when the risk of miscarriage is at its highest. Some couples wait until after the first ultrasound scan, which is sometimes scheduled as early as seven or eight weeks into the pregnancy. If a couple has had a difficult time conceiving or a history of miscarriage, they may choose to wait until the 20-week ultrasound is complete, although concealing the pregnancy for that long may be difficult.

Regardless of what you and your partner end up deciding, it is vital for you to be in total agreement about when and how you will make the announcement. You may want to tell a few close friends and family members in person first, then make a blanket social media announcement to everyone else. Or perhaps you are a little more old-fashioned and wish to make an announcement at a particular party or send out a mail announcement to your family members and friends. Regardless of how you do it, make sure you ask your partner's permission before telling anyone the good news outside of your plan.

## Symptoms of the First Trimester

In many ways, the first trimester can be the most difficult of the three. The physical symptoms can be at their worst due to the rapid increase in hormones that starts immediately after conception. Miscarriages most commonly occur during these first 13 or 14 weeks, so your partner may be filled with anxiety. Besides the hormone-induced emotions, you are both adjusting to the anticipation of becoming parents as well. You'll score extra points by being extra supportive and helpful as she experiences the highs and lows of this trimester.

You already learned all the possible first-trimester physical symptoms, and how you can be supportive and helpful, in Chapter 2. Refer to this list of symptoms now to review and remind yourself that your partner has not turned into a grumpy, unpredictable monster – she's just at the mercy of her body's hormones right now. Go easy on her if she's a little off-kilter, both emotionally and physically, right now.

Though your partner is feeling yucky, this is (once again) your chance to shine. You can treat her and make her feel special in a lot of simple ways at this challenging stage. Come home with a little gift, like baby socks or food she's been craving. Give her a pregnancy massage, along with some lovely oils to battle stretch marks, or get a good DVD for the night. If she bites your head off for your efforts, don't take it personally! Just try again next week.

## Helping Her Eat for Two

The term "eating for two" is a bit misleading, and it often makes women feel like they have permission to eat enough for two full-grown people. However, your partner's nutritional needs will undoubtedly increase over the next nine months, and it is partly your job to help make sure she healthily meets those needs. Healthcare professionals currently recommend that women gain between 25 and 35 pounds during a healthy pregnancy. These recommendations vary based on a woman's starting weight, so be sure she consults her doctor for a personalized recommendation.

On a side note, now is most certainly *not* the time to make any comments about your partner's weight, body size, or food choices. She is more emotionally vulnerable than she has ever been, and you may land yourself permanently in the dog house with one ill-chosen comment or "helpful" suggestion. The best thing you can do is help shop for and prepare healthy food choices, make sure she gets her prenatal vitamins, and be unconditionally loving and supportive. You can encourage her to eat well by setting a good example and laying off the unhealthy options yourself. There's nothing worse than tempting a pregnant woman with food she can't or shouldn't have.

During pregnancy, your partner is literally "making the baby" – in an assembly kind of way – so good ingredients are essential for a quality end product. This means that your unborn baby needs good food. Your partner also needs proper nutrition to help her deal with the physical, mental, and emotional changes and challenges she faces until the baby is born. The female body requires about 10 to 12 percent more energy when she is pregnant. Below are some of the basic nutritional requirements you should help her meet on a daily basis:

- **Six servings of fruits and vegetables:** An apple or tomato is a serving; so is half a cup of salad. Leafy green vegetables are particularly useful as they contain folic acid (see information below), which helps prevent congenital disabilities such as spina bifida.

- **Six servings of grains:** A cup of cooked pasta or rice, or a slice of wholegrain bread or a bread roll makes a serving. Whole grains are particularly useful because they, too, contain folic acid.

- **Three servings of dairy:** A large glass of milk, a small container of yogurt, or two slices of cheese. Low-fat or skim dairy products can help control weight gain.

- **Two servings of protein:** An egg, two slices of lean red meat, or two chicken drumsticks are one serving. Vegetarians can also get protein from nuts and seeds, legumes, and tofu.

## Folic Acid and Other Vitamins

Folic acid, also called folate, is a B vitamin that is important to help prevent certain congenital disabilities. Eating folate-rich foods such as whole grains, chickpeas, and leafy green vegetables helps your partner reach the recommended daily allowance of 400 micrograms. Most pregnancy healthcare providers recommend upping your partner's folic acid by using vitamin supplements, even before she gets pregnant. Check the recommended amount of folic acid, as some women in a high-risk category need more, and follow your health provider's instructions.

## Foods She Shouldn't Eat

Pregnant women shouldn't eat certain foods because of the risk of bacteria, such as listeria, to which pregnant women and unborn babies are incredibly vulnerable. So be sure you don't give her the following foods during pregnancy:

- Any cooked food that has been in the fridge for more than 12 hours
- Cold deli meats or pate.
- Ready-made salads from the deli or your grocery store's refrigerator section.
- Soft cheeses, like blue, ricotta, and blue vein.
- Sprouted seeds.
- Sushi, unless it only contains vegetables or fully cooked fish.
- Unpasteurized milk.
- Undercooked, or runny, eggs.

Ask your primary care provider, obstetrician, or midwife for a comprehensive list of foods and medications to avoid.

By the end of her pregnancy, your partner may be itching to eat a good bit of brie or sushi again, so a great way to celebrate your baby's birth may be to put together a platter of the things your partner's been missing out on for nine months. Start a "foods to remember after birth" list today!

*You Should Get on the Wagon, Too*
Your partner must avoid all kinds of harmful substances to help keep your baby healthy. Seeing you swigging a beer or inhaling sushi will maker her needlessly cranky and resentful, so show some solidarity and stay away from the same things she must avoid.

# Activities to Avoid

While we're on the topic of things to avoid, you should know about some activities your partner should stay away from while she is pregnant. The following activities are not recommended for pregnant women:

- Exciting theme park rides, because of the acceleration the body experiences during the ride.

- Extreme sports and adventure sports, such as skydiving, bungee jumping, parachuting, and whitewater rafting.
- Traveling on a plane, although this mostly applies at the end of the pregnancy.
- Using permanent hair dye, because of the chemicals used in dyes.

You should ask your doctor for a comprehensive list of activities to avoid.

## What's Going on Inside Her Body?

Your partner will appreciate it if you try to educate yourself about the growth and development of your child inside her body. She'll be touched and grateful to see you take an interest in all the fantastic changes that are taking place. Here, we'll give a summary of your baby's growth during each trimester. You can get a more detailed description of the week-by-week changes if you do some research on medical websites, download a reliable app or two on your cell phone or tablet, or buy a book on fetal growth and development. There is an incredible number of reliable resources out there these days!

Between 6 and 12 weeks of gestational development, your baby grows from around one-quarter of an inch long to around 2 inches in length, which is approximately the length of your little finger. In other words, your baby grows about 800 percent in six weeks; no wonder why your partner is so tired!

During this time, your baby's organs take shape. The heart starts beating at around six weeks. Though neither you nor your partner can feel it yet, your little one is moving around in there. She's floating in amniotic fluid in the amniotic sac. The placenta, a specialized organ that grows inside the uterus during pregnancy, is developing to act as life support for your baby.

Between 6 and 12 weeks, your healthcare provider may order an initial ultrasound scan. This first ultrasound is a pretty big deal for most parents-to-be. You get to see your baby for the first time; granted, you may not initially be able to determine what's what until the ultrasound technician points it out. But it's something you'll never forget.

Unfortunately, early ultrasounds can also pinpoint problems with the pregnancy. This happens in about one in six cases; if something is wrong, your partner may have a spontaneous miscarriage or need to terminate the pregnancy for medical reasons. Your doctor will typically mention this before the scan to prepare you in advance. However, you should take the initiative and talk about this potential scenario with your partner before you have the first scan.

## How to Handle the Worst-Case Scenario

Of course, no one wants to think about the idea that their baby might not survive until birth, but it is a possibility for which you and your partner should prepare yourselves, at least in a small corner of your minds. Should a situation arise in which she has a miscarriage, or the baby has such devastating problems that he is unlikely to survive to birth, you will need to be prepared to process your grief and support your partner through her emotional trauma.

A miscarriage is the death of a baby before 20 weeks gestation. Many women don't even know they're pregnant when they miscarry, but many others lose much-wanted and cherished babies. In the past, people have had the attitude that miscarriages are something to be gotten over, that everything will magically improve if they try for another baby. Fathers in particular, who can often seem withdrawn or uncaring about the loss because men can be more private about the way they deal with grief, are encouraged to "just get over it." But for parents who lose babies, it can often be devastating. You also feel you have to be strong for your partner, and in a sense, you do – you need to advocate for your partner at a time when she's confused, angry, vulnerable, and grieving. But you also need to be empathetic and caring, and one way to do that is to talk openly and honestly about your feelings with your partner. You also need to acknowledge your feelings of loss and sadness, rather than pretend to keep a stiff upper lip.

Having a ceremony or funeral for your lost baby may be comforting and give you a chance to express your grief and let others support you. The service can be anything from a few people lighting a candle to a funeral with a minister. Just do anything that comes naturally to you and your partner. Naming your baby can also help you heal – acknowledging your baby as a real person, not a "loss" or an "it," can help.

If you or your partner have the need to talk to someone outside your family or friends, support is available. You have to ask for it. One site that can offer advice and additional support sources is http://miscarriagesupport.com/.

# Being Aware of Pregnancy Depression

Even though pregnancy is supposed to be a fantastic time of anticipation and joy for a woman, many women experience anxiety, stress, or even depression during this time. Recent studies show that between 14 and 23 percent of women will encounter at least some depression symptoms while expecting a child.

Since depression affects approximately 25 percent of all women at some point in their lives, it only makes sense that this disorder can also affect pregnant women. Unfortunately, many people, including the pregnant woman herself, chalk depression symptoms up to hormonal imbalances, so pregnancy depression can go undiagnosed. If diagnosed correctly, depression can be managed with therapy and sometimes medications. However, if left untreated, depression during pregnancy is dangerous for both the mother and the baby.

Another term for depression during pregnancy is antepartum depression. It is classified as a mood disorder, meaning that it is partially due to changes in brain chemistry. Hormone changes and stressful life situations both can affect the chemicals in a pregnant woman's brain, leading to exacerbated symptoms of depression or anxiety. Without treatment, a woman suffering from antepartum depression might engage in risky behavior, such as eating poorly, lack of self-care, drinking alcohol, smoking, and suicidal behavior. All of these behaviors can lead to a baby with developmental problems, low birth weight, or premature birth. Additionally, babies born to depressed mothers may be less active, less attentive, or more agitated than other babies.

Since it is so critical to catch and treat antepartum depression before any damage is done, it is partly your responsibility to monitor your partner's emotional health. Although she may be riding an emotional rollercoaster due to the hormonal changes in her body, you can watch for a few specific symptoms that may be warning signs of clinical antepartum depression. Talk to her regularly to touch bases with her and see how she's feeling. Ask her to help you in watching for the warning signs.

If you or your partner notice that she has experienced any of the following symptoms for two weeks or more, contact your doctor immediately:

- Loss of interest in any of the activities she usually enjoys.
- Difficulty sleeping; or sleeping too much.
- Having trouble concentrating.
- Continual or persistent sadness.

- Anxiety, fear, or persistent worry.
- Feelings of worthlessness or guilt.
- Changes in her eating habits.
- A pattern of hopeless or suicidal thoughts.

If you see any of those symptoms, you must encourage your partner to talk to a mental health professional and get help immediately, for the sake of her health and your unborn baby's health. Your partner is more likely to experience antepartum depression if she has a family history of depression or other mental illnesses, recent relationship issues (with you or in other significant relationships), a history of pregnancy loss, infertility treatments, any stressful life events, a history of abuse or trauma, or if she is experiencing any current complications in her pregnancy.

Remember, the sooner you encourage your partner to get help, the better off she and your baby will be. Depression can be successfully treated and managed, especially with early recognition and intervention. As the person who knows her better than anyone, you can play a big part in preventing the adverse effects of this mood disorder.

# Preparing Your Mindset for Fatherhood

Although it may seem that you still have a long way to go until your little bundle of joy arrives, you will be amazed at how quickly the time passes. To keep yourself from scrambling at the last minute, there are a lot of things you can be doing right now to begin getting ready for your little one. One of the main things you can start doing now is preparing your heart and mind for the idea of becoming a father.

You have probably already begun to realize that your life is about to change forever. You may have had a great relationship with your father, and you might have plenty of friends who have already had a few children, but this will be your first shot at taking on this role yourself. There are many misconceptions about being a father out there, so talk to some people who have experienced the real deal to find out what it's like. Although every father's experience is different, you can start by spending some time with friends who have recently had a baby. If possible, talk to your parents as well.

You must begin to understand that being a father is a lot about acceptance and going with the flow. A useful mantra to remember is "this too shall pass," as every illness, teething episode, a period of sleep deprivation, or colic will pass. Looking after a baby teaches you a lot about life, and you may find that you're more relaxed, confident, and happy as a result of having a child.

Parenting, for both fathers and mothers, requires a certain amount of letting go. When a baby is born, we want things for our child: The best of everything, and every opportunity and good thing in life that may come her way. You naturally want her to avoid the mistakes you made in your own life. But it doesn't always work that way.

Your baby is her own person. She will grow up to have her own ideas, her own interests, and her own strengths, and they may be vastly different from yours. You may want her to be a lawyer, so she has money to pay for things you could only dream of, but what makes her happy is working with animals or in a charity. Sometimes you just have to admit that father *doesn't* know best. You may be disappointed, but it's her life, and only she can live it. Support her; that's what great dads are for.

## Accepting and Embracing Inevitable Changes

Becoming a father is about changing your state of mind and changing the idea of what's important to you. As a dad, the car is less about the ultimate drive and more about keeping your child safe and fitting the stroller in the back.

Besides the car, here are some things that will inevitably change with parenthood:

- **Your work:** If you want to spend time with your family, you may consider working fewer hours or switching to a flexible working arrangement that you can negotiate with your employer. You may even decide to give up work and be the primary caregiver to your child, making you a stay-at-home dad. Remember that dads, just as much as moms, should take part in the day-to-day care of a child.

- **Your freedom:** Doing things when and where you want doesn't work when you have a baby. If the swell is perfect and you feel like going out for a surf, you may have to wait until the baby is asleep or take him and mom along with you. It's the same with spending time out and about with your partner. Going out to dinner and a movie is no longer a spontaneous activity; it requires planning. Finding time for yourself alongside work and family commitments is one of the biggest challenges that fathers face.

- **Your finances:** If you both had an income before your child came along, you'd be down to only one income for a while. If you lived in a one-bedroom apartment, it's time to find something bigger and a way to pay for it.

- **Your friends and family:** Your relationship with friends and family will change. If you live away from your parents, you'll probably find yourself having to spend a lot more time traveling to visit them more often. Some of your childless friends will embrace you having a child and will become the fun "aunt" or "uncle" your child gets excited about seeing. Others will not be so keen on kids, even yours, and you'll see them less as a result.

- **Your vacations:** Going on vacation takes on a whole new meaning. You'll have to postpone that backpacking trip around South America for a few years, at least until your kids are big enough to trudge alongside you. Family vacations are different – great fun, but unlike any vacation you've had since you were a child.

- **Your lifestyle:** Risky lifestyle or sport activities like base jumping or free climbing are no longer just about risking your own life. You now have to consider the future of your child and family.

- **Your health and behavior:** A child is one of the ultimate reasons to change some unhealthy habits like smoking, heavy drinking, eating junk food, and being a slob. Children need a smoke-free environment to breathe in, good healthy food, clean clothes and diapers, and good hygiene to prevent illness. And who needs to grow up hearing foul language?

Sometimes you can plan when you have a child; sometimes nature has her ideas. Either way, fatherhood is a big deal. It's not the same as buying an article of clothing or getting a new plant. Your child, if you decide to have one, has only one shot at life, and he deserves the best opportunity possible. A committed, involved, and reliable father is a big part of that.

If your partner is already pregnant, but you don't feel ready for fatherhood, you've got some time on your side. In the coming months, as your baby grows and gets ready for birth, spend some time with other people's children, talk to other fathers, and let yourself ease into the idea of fatherhood. Think about the kind of father your dad is and what you've learned from him. Think of all the things you would like to do differently.

If you're really, truly not ready for fatherhood as the birth approaches, it may help if you talk to someone about your fears. Your doctor can help you find a counselor. You can find a counselor yourself by looking on the internet but asking other people for recommendations is a better way to find someone who is on your same wavelength. A pastor or other spiritual advisor, if you have one, could be the right person to talk to, or could help you find the right person.

Don't forget to talk to your partner about what you're feeling. After all, you are in this together, so it will help to share your feelings and thoughts with her. She is counting on you to be her teammate in this parenting adventure, so she needs to hear about your thoughts and fears.

# Improving Your Partner's Pregnancy Experience

Even the easiest pregnancy has its difficult times. Starting in this first trimester, you can be educating yourself about what's going on in your partner's body, and then help her get through it in some or all of the following ways:

## Take Care of Your Partner

Growing a baby is hard work, and it takes quite a physical toll on a woman's body. It's true that some women climb mountains until they give birth, but those women are unusual. Some pregnancy symptoms can be completely debilitating for some women. Carrying around all that blood, fluid, and an extra person puts all sorts of strains on your partner's body. Look after your partner continually if necessary, and do everything possible to improve life for her.

## Give Your Partner Some Time Alone

The role of motherhood is quite overwhelming, and your partner is likely experiencing all kinds of mixed emotions about it. For starters, she may be feeling somewhat fearful, as well as exhausted at the mere thought of all the work she must put in over the next 18 years. The least you can do is let her take some time to relax and indulge in some self-care from time to time during pregnancy.

## Attend Medical Appointments with Her

A significant way of showing your support and interest in the pregnancy and your unborn child is by going along to all medical appointments. This way, you and your partner can share the first time you hear your baby's heartbeat or see her moving on the ultrasound scan. Memories like these are irreplaceable.

Going to appointments also supports your partner because, in the event of any unwelcome news, you'll be there to support her.

## Show Excitement over Impending Fatherhood

You may have many fears and reservations about becoming a dad, and your partner may share some of these concerns. However, pretending that the pregnancy doesn't exist will not help. You can talk through any concerns you feel, but you also need to take the time to anticipate all the good things about fatherhood too. If you show some excitement, your partner will be able to relax and show her own excitement, too.

A lot of parenting is about attitude. An anecdote about dealing with picky eaters    sums this up. One father complains that his daughter is a terrible eater and won't eat anything unless it has cheese on it. He's stressed out about it and is pulling his hair out thinking of a solution. On the other hand, another father happily tells    the first guy that his son is a terrific eater because as long as it has cheese on it, he'll eat anything. It's all about attitude!

## Celebrate!

In just a few months, your life will change forever. You'll have to say goodbye to much of the spontaneity and freedom that characterized your earlier adult life and take on a lot of responsibility. For now, you should take advantage of the time you have left with just your partner and take her on plenty of dates.

One dad-to-be surprised his partner with a picnic lunch at the local zoo in the weeks before their baby was born. He'd even packed sparkling grape juice to toast their health and a pillow for his partner to sit on. She spent most of her time waddling back and forth from the restroom, but the gesture was most appreciated.

# Chapter 4: Enjoying the Second, or "Golden" Trimester

The second trimester is sometimes called the "golden trimester," because the initial symptoms of morning sickness and sheer exhaustion usually wane, your partner starts to feel more energy, and she hasn't yet started to suffer the discomforts of the third trimester. Because she is feeling better, your partner may begin to take on the expected pregnancy "glow." This trimester is marked by weeks 14 through 28 of pregnancy.

## The First Kicks and the Baby Bump

During the second trimester, you'll start to see your partner's body change more as the baby grows. The baby bump, if it hasn't already made an appearance, will become more evident as this trimester progresses. As your partner's belly is getting bigger, the reality that you're going to have a child may start to set in for you. Exciting times!

Sometime in the second trimester, your partner will also probably start feeling those first kicks and bumps. This typically happens around 18 to 20 weeks, but she may not recognize them at first, especially if this is her first pregnancy. Some women may not notice the movements of their first baby until closer to weeks 22 through 24. Eventually, you'll be able to feel the movements from outside her belly, too. They may be hard to spot at first, as that little foot tries to get in touch with you through all those abdominal muscles. Feeling those kicks for the first time is a pretty magical moment for dads-to-be.

# Common Side Effects in the Second Trimester

Most side effects that your partner will experience during this trimester are results of the growing size of your baby. They include the following:

## Back Pain

This symptom is perhaps one of the most common complaints of pregnant women and is caused by the growing weight of the baby, additional strain on the spine, and a change in the center of gravity that the body needs to adjust for. You will be a superstar if you offer her lots of backrubs (use as much or as little pressure as she prefers) with or without massage oils or lotions. Give her plenty of opportunities to relax in any position that is comfortable for her or take hot baths to ease the pain in her back. She may feel relief from laying on a heating pad, too. Laying directly on her back is not recommended as her baby grows, because it can reduce circulation to the baby. You can help her get comfortable on her side, with a hot water bottle or heating pad against her aching back.

## Constipation

This is a common problem during pregnancy. The main reason for constipation in the second trimester is an increase in the hormone progesterone, which slows the movement of food through the digestive tract. Later in pregnancy, the problem of constipation is likely to be made worse by the pressure of the growing uterus on the intestines. Taking iron supplements, which many pregnant women take, can also make constipation worse. You can help by encouraging her by going for easy-to-moderately-paced strolls to aid digestion, preparing foods rich in fiber, like green leafy vegetables and whole grains, and asking your partner's healthcare provider if she recommends stool softening medications or enemas. It's certainly not an enjoyable topic to discuss, but you'll be her hero if you can help in any way!

## Heartburn

This burning sensation in the middle chest is caused by the hormone progesterone, which softens the esophagus, allowing acid to come back out. So, if your partner complains about heartburn, don't be offended – your cooking probably isn't the cause! You can offer a glass of milk or some bread to see if it helps reduce the burning. Sometimes, sleeping with her upper body elevated can also ease the pain so you can help prop her up with extra pillows at night. If this symptom becomes severe, there are some safe medications that she can take during pregnancy, so talk to her healthcare provider about possible prescriptions if the need arises.

## Leg cramps

These seem to plague pregnant women more at night. They can arise due to a variety of factors, including decreased circulation in the legs (thanks to the baby resting on blood vessels). Fatigue or the uterus putting pressure on nerves might also be to blame. Finally, a deficiency of magnesium or calcium, or simple dehydration, might cause these pains. You can offer to gently (or firmly, if she prefers) massage the cramps, even when they occur in the wee hours of the morning. She may be eternally grateful if you help her into a warm Epsom salt bath, too. Help her make sure she is taking in enough proper nutrition and drinking plenty of water. If nothing is helping, talk to her doctor to see if she has additional recommendations.

## Softening ligaments

The ligaments in the pelvis stretch, which widens the pelvis to prepare for birth. It can give your partner a floating sensation in the joints and cause sharp stabbing pains when she stands up to quickly or rolls over in bed. This is called round ligament pain, and it is a good sign that your partner's body is making the right adjustments in preparation for the birth. Help ease her pain by reminding her to take it slow when standing up or sitting down and offer plenty of sympathies when she is struck by a sudden sharp pain.

Other than the specific suggestions for each symptom, you can also continue to offer lots of support, love, and encouragement to your partner.

# What's Going on Inside Her Body?

At 24 weeks, your baby is nearly 12 inches long, or about the length from your elbow to your wrist! She is also busy going through these fantastic developments:

## Developing her eyes

Pigmentation in the iris (the colored part of the eye) develops. If your baby is of European descent, she'll be born with blue eyes that may change color in the months after birth. African American, Native American, and Asian babies can be born with brown or blue eyes, and eye color can also change with time.

## Covered in moisturizer

Your baby's using the world's best moisturizer, vernix, a waxy coating that keeps her skin from getting wrinkled as she floats around in fluid all day. She's also growing fingernails, hair, and eyebrows.

## Beginning to distinguish sounds

Your baby can hear now but won't know what she hears for a long time yet. However, research suggests that babies recognize their parents' voices when they're born from what they hear in the womb. Amazing, isn't it?

## Almost done with the major structures

By the end of the second trimester, your baby is almost done growing and developing all external and internal organs.

Again, your partner will be touched and grateful if you try to keep learning about all the incredible changes your baby is going through as he grows and develops inside her body.

## Medical Things You Should Know

Because 80 percent of miscarriages happen in the first 12 weeks, many parents don't announce their pregnancy until the second trimester. Now is also the time to ask about a nuchal fold test to check for potential congenital disabilities, especially if your partner is age 35 or older. A nuchal fold test aims to determine the likelihood of your baby being born with Down syndrome. Your healthcare provider might also suggest alternative tests, such as a blood test for DNA screening, to help determine the likelihood of genetic disorders in your baby. Make sure you ask a lot of questions about any tests that are recommended, so you understand your options and any risk factors involved with the tests. Remember, you and your partner are the ones paying the bill here, so you are in charge of the care that she and your baby get!

Around 20 weeks, your midwife, obstetrician, or family doctor may send you for an ultrasound scan to make sure that the baby's development is on track and that things are progressing smoothly. The 20-week scan is a significant milestone, and you'll probably get to go home with a DVD of pictures or even videos of your little one! If you can't wait another 20 weeks to find out your baby's sex, you can usually find out at this scan, unless junior has his legs crossed! Some of the DNA scans mentioned in the previous section have the bonus of revealing your baby's sex if you would like to find out before the birth.

You should also know that sex during pregnancy is okay in most cases (ask your doctor) and is even good for the baby as well. The second trimester may be the best time to share a bit of passion, although it depends on how your partner is feeling throughout pregnancy. By the way, it's not out of the question to have sex almost up until labor, depending on how your partner feels. Always remember to be sensitive to her moods. Even if it has been a long dry spell for you, she may be thoroughly exhausted or too uncomfortable for sex. Just imagine trying to enjoy sex while your esophagus feels as if it's on fire, you haven't had a bowel movement in a week, your back aches, and you keep having random leg cramps! Be patient; she'll feel better eventually.

## Continuing to Improve Your Partner's Experience

Now that you're safely in the second trimester and your partner is (hopefully) feeling less sick than in the previous trimester, there are some additional things you can do to help her celebrate and enjoy this time.

### Go on a "Babymoon"

Before you are saddled with a little one, now is a perfect time to take a relaxing vacation together. Although common pregnancy sense dictates that you shouldn't go to any developing nations, and plane travel may not be recommended, there are plenty of luxurious places you can visit within the good old United States.

### Learn and Prepare with Her

Your partner will be excited and appreciative to see you educating yourself about baby knowledge and skills. There is a lot to learn, so why not throw yourself into the process? You can find out about prenatal classes in your area, for starters.

## Record That Beautiful Belly

Centuries and even decades ago, the iconic pregnant belly was hidden as if it was something shameful. Now, you can help your partner feel more attractive, while simultaneously documenting the changes your baby is going through under the surface, by taking regular pictures of the baby bump. You can even consider hiring a professional photographer. Those who are practiced in maternity photography can help her appreciate her new shape and regain some confidence.

# Beginning to Shop for Baby

You see your partner transform as the baby grows, and she may start planning what to buy (not more clothes!) and how to decorate the baby's room. This is called "the nesting instinct," and you pretty much have to go with it. When it comes to buying things for the baby, however, dads are hugely important as they tend to "keep it real." Many household budgets are under a lot of pressure when the baby arrives, and with your partner being high on hormones, you should go shopping together to avoid a local financial crisis. See the next chapter for an overview of what you need to buy.

# Chapter 5: Home Preparations

Few things change the way you live as much as welcoming a baby into your life. Having a baby is like having a house guest who never cleans up after himself, cries a lot, and has more needs than you and your partner put together. Adding a baby to the family is not as simple as clearing out the spare room for him to sleep in. He needs stuff: clothes, bedding, diapers, all sorts of things you need to think about that become part of your daily life as a father.

As you count down to your baby's birth, you need to get things done to avoid hassles down the line – get those bags packed and ready for the hospital, get the bassinet and a car seat sorted out, and be prepared to go at a moment's notice. When he arrives, the chances are that you won't have a lot of time for decorating the baby's room or shopping for socks, so it's best to get those things out of the way now.

In decades past, preparing for the baby was thought of as primarily the woman's domain. The future mother alone was responsible for doing all the shopping and decorating the baby's room. However, this responsibility is split between partners more and more, and you will find that your partner, who is becoming more fatigued and weighed down by your growing bundle of joy each day, will be eternally grateful for any contributions you make to the preparation process.

In this chapter, you'll discover the ins and outs of what to look for when buying things like nursery furniture, strollers, diapers, clothes, and toys. You'll find out what a diaper rash is, how to prevent it, and how to help your baby when he's teething. You'll get checklists for everything you need to do before the birth and what you need to take with you to the hospital or have prepared for a home birth.

The point of all this information is so you can share as equally as possible in the process of getting ready for your precious little one. Your partner has taken the lion's share of the work by growing your child inside her body, so it's time for you to step up, roll up your sleeves, and get excited about shopping for baby stuff!

## Getting the Right Gear

Who would have thought a baby would need so much stuff? Getting set up for a new person in your house takes a bit of thought – and a mountain of cash if you're not careful. Rather than telling you to go out and buy every bit of gear, the baby shops say you absolutely must have; this guide will tell you what you need.

First, to keep costs down, send the word around among your coworkers and friends that you're having a baby. They may have cribs, bassinets, car seats, and strollers they're no longer using. You can completely outfit a nursery for very little or even for free if you have generous friends and relatives.

# The Overwhelming World of Baby Clothes

Baby clothes come in more shapes and styles than you would have thought possible. Babies don't dress like miniature adults. They hate itchy materials, fussy buttons, and other things you might put up with to be fashionable. However, because adults and not babies buy clothes, you'll find a whole spectrum of cute stuff specifically designed to appeal to adults, covered with duckies and little toy cars.

## Types of Baby Clothes

Be forewarned – it's hard to resist this stuff, especially for moms-to-be. But check out what works for you before you break the bank.

- **Bodysuits** are long- or short-sleeved T-shirts that also cover the baby's diaper area and snap at the bottom for easy changing. They are handy for keeping everything tucked in, so that baby's tummy doesn't get chilly, and they also keep him looking pulled together. They're great during the summer months when a short-sleeved bodysuit can be worn by itself without pants or as pajamas.

- **Footies** are all-in-one outfits that either snap or zip up the legs and front. They're like bodysuits with leg coverings and socks. Some snap up the back, which is inconvenient. Most have feet, but you can get some without feet (called "nonfooties" or "coveralls") for summer. Most also have long sleeves.

- **Sleeping bags** (also called gowns) are like footies with sleeves but no legs, just a sack covering your baby's legs and feet. The American Academy of Pediatrics recommends not using blankets in cribs for infants up to one year, so having her wear a sleeping bag will help her stay warm. Gowns that have elastic around the bottom are also fabulous for late-night diaper changes because if her legs are bare under the sack, you can get to the diaper more easily and disturb her less.

## Listing the Clothes Your Baby Needs

The following list is a guide for things you should have ready to go for your newborn baby. You can customize your list as you figure out which items work well for you. You can also tweak the list to suit the seasons. In general, baby clothes should be loose-fitting, made with breathable and soft fabric, not too tight at the neck, and easy to open and close. Keep in mind that you can go through three to four outfits a day because of diaper leaks and baby spit-up. Here's a general idea of what you need:

- **Plenty of bodysuits:** You'll need at least six, probably more.

- **Four footies:** As with bodysuits, the more, the better. These are favorite baby shower gifts.

- **Four pairs of pants of some sort:** Overalls are cute, but make sure they have snaps in the legs, so you don't have to take the whole thing off to change a diaper. Elastic waists on pants are far easier than fumbling around with zippers and snaps.

- **Four sleeping bags:** Look for cotton material instead of polar fleece or microfleece, since these fabrics are less breathable and may lead to overheating.

- **Two jackets:** Look for jackets that are easy to zip or snap, since buttons take too long to do up.

- **Two sweaters or wraparound jerseys:** Choose the kinds that don't need to go over her head. Most babies hate having things pulled over their head.

- **Plenty of pairs of socks:** Make them all the same if possible – one is always getting lost.

- **Four hats:** These should be made of a Lycra-cotton mix, so they stretch, or soft wool if they're handmade. Some babies dislike hats and try to pull them off, so look for something that snaps or ties under the chin if necessary.

- **Plenty of bibs with snaps or Velcro:** Bibs with ties can be difficult to put on. Velcro stops sticking after some washings. Some large bibs go on over baby's head.

- **Two pairs of soft shoes:** Typically, shoes that have elastic around the heel stay on better than other slip-ons. Babies don't need real shoes until they're walking outside.

- **Two pairs of gloves or mittens:** It's best to get some that clip to your baby's outerwear because these are lost easily!

## Tips for Selecting Baby Clothes

Here are some tips for selecting clothes, based on the experiences of real babies and parents. Your partner will be thoroughly impressed and relieved at your knowledge of these little insights:

- Avoid anything that doesn't have a few snaps at the shoulder or an envelope-style neckband, to make pulling the clothing over her face painless.
- Avoid anything that has a back opening. Your baby will inevitably spend a lot of time laying on her back in early months, and it can't be comfortable to have snaps under you. They're also tricky to get on when you're getting her dressed.
- Avoid anything that looks like it's going to be a pain to put on. Some babies hate the process of getting dressed, and trying

to tie silly ribbons when she's having a meltdown isn't anyone's idea of a good time.

- If your baby arrives in the winter, look for clothes that have folds sewn into the ends of the sleeves. These are mittens. They're also great for keeping your baby from scratching himself with those sharp newborn nails.
- If in doubt about sizing, buy clothes that are too big. At least you know junior will grow into them. Avoid the newborn or 0-3 month sizes, unless your baby is tiny or a preemie.
- If you've been given a lot of hand-me-down clothing, be aware that the fire retardant in some clothing may be worn and will not be as effective as it is in new clothes.
- You will be given a ton of new clothing as presents, so if you find you have too much, don't be afraid to take it back to the store and exchange it for something you can use in the future, like the next size up.
- Dark colors show baby spit-up much more than light colors, but light colors show baby poop much more! Just go with the colors you like.
- Handling a baby in the first few months can feel a bit tricky because she can

appear fragile. Think about what steps you need to go through to put on an item of clothing. If it seems too complicated to close or open an item, don't buy it.

- When trying to determine what size your baby needs, try to go by the weight chart provided by the manufacturer. The months listed as sizes usually have very little to do with your baby's age.

## Filling the Toy Box

When your baby is born, all he does for a while is poop, pee, eat, cry, sleep, and gaze at things with an unfocused stare. So, he won't need electronic gear, a racing car set, or a mini piano just yet. What he needs are things that give him a real sense of the world he's just come into – simple objects that provide new sights, shapes textures, smells, sounds, and sensations.

You can quickly provide all these characteristics just by spending time with your baby, singing to him, and touching his skin and fingers with textures like an old comb, fabric, your hair, leaves, the cat's fur, etc. As he begins to grasp and bring his hands together, things like a rattle or a chain of plastic rings can keep him fascinated for a long time.

When your baby starts teething, he looks for things to put in his mouth to push against his gums to relieve the discomfort. Many toys would double as teething rings, even if they weren't initially designed for this purpose.

Here are some good ideas for baby toys:

- **Cloth or hard cardboard books:** Look for ones with flaps or things to touch sewn into them so your baby can experience different textures. Reading to your child every day is one of the most important gifts you can give him.

- **Plastic keys:** For some reason, babies love your car keys, so give them their own set! These are great for teething too. However, nearly every baby will still prefer your keys to his, so keep yours out of his reach.

- **Play gyms:** These are mats with arms curved over the top where you can attach bright objects like soft toys or musical objects for your baby to look at as he lies on the mat. Just make sure he can't pull down anything that he shouldn't be chewing on. Nothing is safe from his gummy mouth once he's got the hang of his hands.

- **Rattles:** You can buy rattles or make your own from old plastic containers filled with noisy objects. Ensure the lid is on securely and never leave your baby alone with an object that could come apart.

- **Soft toy animals:** One of these will probably become your baby's most treasured friend, and it will never be the one you favor, so only guy stuffed animals you won't mind seeing for the next six years. Avoid button eyes and other removable parts a baby could choke on.

Remember, you probably don't need a whole lot when it comes to toys, no matter what the manufacturers tell you. Nothing beats spending time playing and exploring with your baby. Brain development is assisted by appropriate stimulation and human contact.

To make sure toys are safe for your little one, check for any parts that may become a choking hazard and toxins, such as toxic paints. Inevitably your little guy will try to put all toys (and most other things) into his mouth, so make sure they're safe to put in his mouth.

## Stroller Shopping

Strollers have evolved quite a bit since you were a child. These days, many strollers will fit together with your baby's first car seat. As a result, you can transfer the whole seat into the stroller without removing him when he's a newborn.

Baby stores are often packed with different models of strollers. This item is often one of the most significant purchases you make in the parenthood game, so take your time when shopping around.

Here are some features you should search for:

- Can the car seat attach to it? Many brands make travel systems with integrates strollers and car seats.
- Does the stroller include a fitted sunshade and weather cover?
- How easy is it to move the stroller through store doors, the doors of your house, and fold it for storage?
- How easy is it to adjust the back of the seat?
- Is the stroller rugged enough to take off-road on unpaved walkways and trails?

## Choosing the Right Car Seat

Using a car seat for your most precious cargo is not optional. You may have free-ranged in your parents' car when you were little and lived to tell the tale, but sadly some children haven't survived. So, make sure you always use a car seat when traveling with your baby.

As with strollers, so many models of car seats are out there that it pays to shop around. There are different sizes according to the age and weight of your child. For the first model that you purchase, you want to search specifically for an infant car seat or a convertible infant car seat. An infant car seat is specifically used for newborns up to approximately 20 pounds or more. Many infant car seats snap handily into a base that you install into the car ahead of time using seatbelts. For the utmost safety reasons, infants should be kept in rear-facing car seats until they reach the weight limit of the rear-facing seat or are at least two years old.

 Feeding, Bathing, and Entertaining

You thought you were done shopping in the baby aisle? Oh no – there's much more to fill up your house with! You'll find most of these things lurking in homes where children live:

- **Baby bathtub:** You need something to wash your baby in. The kitchen sink may work just fine for a while, but he'll eventually need something a bit larger, but not as large as the regular bathtub. Changing tables that converted to infant baths used to be common, but many parents don't have the room for them. If you do have one, it'll save some wear and tear on your back. Otherwise, you'll need something to set in the big bathtub, at least until your baby can sit up by himself. A bath support is a ramp that baby can lie back on that holds her at a 45-degree angle, so her head is safely kept out of the water. There are many different styles, and you and your baby may prefer one type to another, so shop around.

- **Bouncy chair or infant seat:** Most kids have spent time in a bouncy chair or infant seat, which is a baby chair that your baby can lie in to watch you go about your day from a better angle than lying on the floor. These seats are portable and easy to clean, and she can even sit outside in one while you're gardening. Some have built-in vibrating mechanisms that calm a fussy baby, while others have activity trays that keep baby busy period these seats come with safety straps that should be used every time you put the baby in it.

- **High chair:** When your baby starts solids, you're going to need somewhere she can sit to be fed. A wide range of high chair models is available, from chairs with an ergonomic design made of wood that hasn't been treated with chemicals to chairs with more levers and straps than a space shuttle. Having a detachable tray that you can take off and clean regularly is essential, as are safety straps so you can be sure she isn't going to wriggle her way out of it and get hurt. As an alternative to a high chair, you may want to use a model that attaches to your table. Later on, you can use a little booster seat that you strap to a normal chair.

- **Swing:** No, this isn't the kind of swing you can attach to the apple tree. This kind lives inside your house and takes up about half your living room. Baby swings can be lifesavers if you have a fussy baby because the constant movement suits him, although watching it may drive you crazy.

## Making Room for the Baby

When you were growing up, do you remember how important your bedroom was? It's more than a place where a child's bed is or where his clothes are stored. It's a child sanctuary, his own special space that has all the things he loves close by. Although he won't know this for a while yet, you can start creating that individual, happy space for him before he's born. But first, we cover what every nursery needs to have. Your partner will be especially appreciative of all your efforts to help get the nursery ready. Although she may have the final say in the décor and how the furniture is arranged, you can help by making sure you have everything you need and by putting everything together for her. By doing all the heavy lifting and other manual labor, you're letting her rest and focus on her most important task – growing your baby.

## Finding Functional Furniture and Gear

Here are the essential items you should get for your baby's nursery:

- **A place to sleep:** Many parents prefer to place their children in a bassinet for the first few months of their lives. Eventually, they will sleep in a crib, where they will stay until about 2 years of age. If you decide to get a used crib, be sure to research current safety recommendations for crib bars and mattresses.

- **A changing table:** You should look for a changing table that has the option of a strap to buckle around your little one when he starts rolling and twisting. The best changing table pads have washable covers and waterproof liners. It's also best to find a changing table that has drawers, so you can easily reach any essential supplies while changing the diaper.

- **A dresser or closet (or both);** Although infant clothes are tiny, they end up taking up a lot of room! Since you'll want to have multiple sizes on hand for rapid growth, you will probably fill up a small infant dresser or standard-sized closet quickly. It may benefit both you and your partner to come up with an organizational system for storing clothes of different sizes, especially if you are given a lot of hand-me-down clothes.

- **Other basic essentials:**
  - A diaper pail with a pedal for hands-free opening.
  - A rocking chair or glider where either parent can feed the baby. As the baby grows, you can read pre-bedtime stories and share cuddles in this chair, too.
  - A bookshelf or toy box.
  - Toiletries like diaper cream, wipes, and powder.
  - All recommended health items, like nail clippers, a thermometer, children's liquid acetaminophen, and a snot sucker.

## Decorating the Nursery

Decorating your baby's room is another way to clean out your wallet in a hurry, as there are thousands of things to put in a little person's room to add personality and style. Expectant moms have been known to get carried away so you may have to display a bit of good old male shopping rationale. Babies spend a lot of time gazing into space when they're really small, as if they're tuning into a radio show you can't hear, and like looking at high-contrast objects around them, such as black and white shapes. Keep the decorating simple. As your baby develops his taste and his needs change, transforming the nursery into a little child's room won't take a complete overhaul.

Here are some tips for keeping the decorations simple:

- Keep the colors and designs neutral, so that the room can easily be redecorated as your baby grows.
- Use pictures of close friends and family on the wall so your baby can grow up knowing who the important people are.
- Mobiles hanging from the ceiling don't have to be fancy. A string of shells hanging from driftwood can entertain a small baby, but make sure anything you hang is extremely durable, so it doesn't

fall apart on the baby's head. Also, make sure the mobile is well out of a baby's reach because small pieces or hanging strings can be a choking or strangling hazard; remove the mobile when he's able to get to it.

- Use removable decals on the walls so they can be easily taken off as baby grows up and out of the nursery themes. Choose things that won't damage the wallpaper or paint.

There is infinite information out there about physical preparation for a child in your home, so don't let yourself get overwhelmed. Take the advice and information that seem practical and helpful and ignore the rest. You'll eventually learn through trial and error exactly what you need for your unique family and child.

# Chapter 6: The Final Countdown, A.K.A. the Third Trimester

You're on the final lap now. Don't get too excited though; you still have some hoops to jump through.

## Childbirth Education Classes

Start thinking about childbirth education classes, which your care provider can refer you to. These classes can be extremely valuable in terms of educating you about the process of birth, can answer any burning questions you might have and can allow you to meet other prospective dads who are just as excited – or terrified – as you are. Lots of people go on to keep in touch with their classmates as their babies grow. Your hospital probably offers these classes for expectant parents. If you're interested in a certain birthing method, such as the Bradley method, or Lamaze, you may find classes that discuss these birthing types.

Checking with someone who has already attended a prenatal class you are interested in is definitely a good idea. Some classes are more dad-inclusive than others. For example, some providers split the group into moms and dads to talk about specific issues or situations. Having a guys-only session as part of a prenatal class is great, as it provides the ideal opportunity for some "man talk" about pregnancy, babies, and fatherhood.

While most childbirth education or prenatal classes focus on the birth of your baby, it's a good idea to pick up some tips and tricks about getting through the first few weeks and months. Fortunately, there are now many courses available where, as a guy, you feel less awkward. Some are even designed just for dads!

You may wonder whether you really have to go to prenatal classes. The answer is yes! Not necessarily because you learn amazing things, but because your partner appreciates it. Additionally, you can network with other couples and dads who are in the same boat as you.

Class content varies wildly, so try to shop around early if you can and check what's offered before you decide to sign on the dotted line. Apart from the standard options we mentioned earlier, you can also find alternative classes or providers by asking your healthcare provider and checking with your friends who have had babies. Your local hospital will almost always provide some type of class, from labor prep to newborn care skills.

If you want to go beyond the basics of baby and child care, you can also check out courses that teach baby massage, baby sign language, and activities with babies. Your partner will be amazed and impressed at any effort you make to go above and beyond the standard fare of childbirth education. Just think of how much more relaxed and confident she will feel if she sees you taking the initiative and learning to be the best father you can be!

# Making Choices About the Birth

The time has come to start looking forward to The Big Day. That baby is going to have to come out, sooner or later. These days, you're faced with a lot of choices concerning how your little bundle of joy enters the world. Home birth or hospital birth? No drugs, or all the drugs you can get? With lots of family members, a video camera, and updates on Twitter? Or just your partner, the person delivering the baby, and you?

## Pain Relief Options

First up to think about – and possibly foremost in your partner's mind right now – are the pain relief options. There's a swing towards having as little intervention or being as natural and drug-free as possible during labor and birth. But ultimately, the pain relief options really depend on your partner's preferences. Toward the end of pregnancy, she's probably grappling with the idea of what labor is going to be like and the pressure to be as stoic about it as possible. Supporting your partner and standing by whatever decisions she makes regarding her body and the birth of your baby goes a long way toward making it easier on her.

Here's a look at the pain relief options:

- **Drug-free:** Heat packs, massage, breathing exercises, and being in water may help relieve the pain of labor. Keeping active during the birth and avoiding lying on her back can also help your partner manage the pain.

- **Epidural:** An epidural is a local anesthetic injected into the spinal column. It blocks out all pain and is often used during cesareans so the mother can be awake when her child is born. Around 60 percent of American women have epidural anesthesia in labor.

- **Narcotics:** Intravenous pain relievers, including narcotics and sedatives, can cause drowsiness in both mother and baby, though usually without any long-term effects. Most healthcare providers won't give them if they think your partner is close to delivery because they can depress the baby's breathing. They can also cause nausea.

## Where and How to Have the Baby

Another big decision is where and how to have the baby. No doubt your partner has researched all options by now. Unfortunately, the "I just want to wake up in the morning, and my baby will be here" option doesn't exist. She's probably let you know what her next best option is. If she hasn't told you, you should ask her about it.

The most common scenarios are;

- **Birth centers or free-standing birth centers:** Having your baby in a special birth center run by midwives may provide you with additional options to try particular birthing techniques or varying positions during labor. However, birth centers generally take a non-interventionist approach and don't provide epidurals. And if you need a cesarean section or your baby requires special care, you'll need to be transferred to a hospital.

- **Home birth:** This option has become more popular but is still the exception in the United States. Less than 2 percent of American women give birth at home. For a home birth, you need the support of a midwife, usually a certified or lay midwife, if your state regulations allow because most nurse-midwives deliver in hospitals or birthing centers. If your partner wants a water birth, you can rent special equipment to facilitate the birth at home.

- **Hospital birth:** Most women in the United States opt for a hospital birth. Some hospitals provide extra facilities for water births or natural (as in no pain relief) births.

Talk to your care provider about your options and discuss the pros and cons of each one. Do not be afraid to ask questions and be sure you know everything you need to be confident about the upcoming birth. As your partner's number-one support person, you must know what's going on as much as she does.

Your health insurance may dictate your choice of healthcare providers or even which hospital you use. Check out your policy at the beginning of pregnancy to avoid unwelcome surprises later.

# More Medical Things You Should Know

As you head into the home stretch of pregnancy, you have more checkups with your midwife or obstetrician, and you and your partner may work out a birth plan. This may sound like an oxymoron, as birth is one process to which you just have to surrender, and you have very little control over what happens. Lots of pain relief options and delivery methods are available, so be clear with your midwife or obstetrician about which of these you're interested in and which you're not. That's what a birth plan is – a clear understanding of how you would like things to go so that the person delivering your baby knows your wishes.

Keep an open mind about how the birth will go. If you've planned for a nice water birth at home, be prepared that if things don't go as smoothly as you would like, you may have to be transferred to the hospital. Or if you've said there's absolutely no way your woman needs pain relief, she may be yelling for an epidural in the first five minutes. The ultimate aim is delivering your baby safely into the world with the least amount of anxiety and trauma on your beloved partner so you can set off on your parenting path on the healthiest and safest foot possible.

Your healthcare provider checks the baby's position and makes sure she's in the right place. During this trimester your baby makes her way down headfirst toward the cervix, ready for birth, a process called engaging. If she has her feet pointed down toward the cervix, she's in a breech position. If she stays breech until the birth, the chances are that your care provider will recommend a cesarean birth.

Your caregiver may also take swabs from your partner's vagina to test for *group B strep*, which is a bacteria that can infect your baby as she's being born. This test is often performed during the second half of pregnancy. If traces of it are discovered, your partner will probably need to be on an antibiotic drip during labor.

# Common Side Effects of the Third Trimester

By now, the golden glow of the second trimester may be getting a bit tarnished. As your partner nears her due date, your baby is starting to take over her body – literally! Her internal organs are getting pushed and shoved all over the place, and her abdominal muscles have split in the middle to make way for that wide load she's carrying. Your partner may even waddle already, as her relaxed ligaments widen her pelvis.

Some common complaints during this time include the following:

## "Baby brain"

Pregnant women often feel like they're losing their marbles. They tend to forget things, don't remember simple or frequent activities, and appear to be running around like headless chickens. These symptoms are believed to be caused by hormones, lack of sleep, and the general toll pregnancy takes on the body. Above all else, be sympathetic, understanding, and gentle with your partner. The chances are good that she is more frustrated with her forgetfulness than you are. You can gently remind her when she forgets things, but never appear that you are scolding her or angry. She already feels bad enough.

## Insomnia and fatigue

Insomnia is one thing most mothers-to-be in the third trimester agree on. Her joints may be sore, back aching, with a baby that kicks all night and heartburn to boot. Your partner may also need to get up to urinate every five minutes. Lying on her back to sleep can put pressure on the vena cava, an important artery feeding the heart, so she has to lie on her side at night, and turning over in bed can be a little trying. You can suggest that she try a pillow under her right side, where the vena cava is, which tilts the weight of her body off the artery. You can also help by trying to help her relax. Offer a massage, aromatherapy, or a nice body pillow – basically, anything that might help her drift off to sleep for a few hours would be greatly appreciated!

## Varicose veins – and hemorrhoids!

The third trimester can be hard on a girl. She's getting rounder by the day and may waddle; she's tired, and not getting enough sleep is making her grumpy. And then the hemorrhoids turn up and make her feel downright miserable. She's not feeling like a radiant mother-to-be anymore; she's feeling like a veiny, fat frump. Varicose veins and piles can be raised or made worse by the weight of the baby on her body, so get her to take it easy and rest a lot. Keep doing the lion's share of the housework. The less she has to do, the more rested she'll be for the impending labor. And keep reminding her of how beautiful she is to you.

## Fluid retention

As well as carrying a rapidly growing baby around, your partner's retaining fluid and has more blood flowing through her body. In hot weather or after standing for long periods, this blood collects in her ankles. Your partner should put her feet up whenever she can and avoid salty foods. A few foot rubs from dad would be welcome, too. Keep in mind that any joking comments about her size or appearance will likely have you sleeping in the doghouse for the rest of your natural life – and you will deserve it.

## Varying tastes and cravings

That pesky hormone progesterone causes unusual food cravings, along with all the other bothersome symptoms that it causes. Finding anything that tastes just how she wants it may be very hard for your partner, and predicting what she needs is almost impossible. Try to just roll with it and keep up your partner's spirits by suggesting lots of different options.

Taking slow walks together, reading or singing to the baby in bed at night, making lists of potential names together, and taking photos of the growing baby bump makes for a good time and help you support each other as the big day approaches. These are some of your last days before your family numbers grow, so take time to be with your partner right now. She will look back and cherish the memories of these days together.

# What's Going on Inside Her?

Your baby is just putting on the finishing touches before making his glorious entry into the world. He's been keeping busy with the following critical developments:

## Gaining weight

At the start of the third trimester, your baby weighed about 2 pounds, but by the end, he has reached his birth weight – between 7.5 and 8 pounds, on average. At just 32 weeks, he is already 16 to 17 inches long, which is almost as long as he will be at birth. Now he just needs to pack on some weight. The most rapid weight gain – half a pound per week – happens in the final few weeks.

## Getting in position

In most cases, your baby is head down with his feet under your partner's rib cage. No wonder she's uncomfortable! If your baby is butt down, he's in a breach position, which could necessitate a cesarean section. But babies can and do turn into the vertex, or head-down position, any time in pregnancy. After 36 weeks, it becomes less likely, due to the cramped space.

## Practicing for life on the outside

Your baby is taking practice breaths and urinating into the amniotic fluid. His eyes are open, and you may see him holding the umbilical cord or sucking his thumb on ultrasound scans.

## Naming Your Little One

One topic that you and your partner may have already discussed at length is the name you are going to call junior when he or she makes an appearance. Perhaps you already know your child's gender and have the perfect name all picked out. Or maybe you're waiting to find out your baby's sex at birth, and you have a couple of different names in mind. Or perhaps you're just waiting to meet your baby face-to-face before you decide on a name that best suits her. Either way, make sure you are on the same page with your partner when it comes to naming your sweet baby. The name of your child is certainly not worth an intense argument; if you find that you have very different opinions about names, there is always a way to compromise. For example, if your partner has her mind set on a family name that you find unappealing, perhaps you could compromise by using it as the child's middle name.

As with all other things in pregnancy, keeping the lines of communication open while expressing emotions calmly will go a way towards helping keep the peace. Remember, your partner is under a lot of stress and the influence of some crazy hormones. You need to maintain a sense of calm and rationality to help lower her stress levels.

## Helping Her Make Decisions About Work

Your partner may be facing a difficult decision or two when it comes to employment as you count down the days before the arrival of your baby. Some women find themselves torn about how much time to take off work and whether they will be returning to work at all after the addition of a new family member. There is no right or wrong way to approach these decisions, and you must remember to be sensitive to the possibility that she might change her mind after she has spent a few weeks with the new baby.

Finances and employment benefits often weigh heavily towards making decisions about length of maternity leave and whether your partner will return to work or become a stay-at-home mother. She may have already made up her mind about how long she will be off work, and she may have no trouble at all when it comes to sticking to this decision. However, some women struggle intensely with the idea of leaving their babies after they have spent a week or two caring for them. They may have initially decided to enroll your newborn in daycare, but they may ultimately decide that they are more comfortable with the idea of staying home for the first year or two of your child's life.

Unless you are blessed with close friends or family members who will care for the baby free of charge, daycare is often very costly. You and your partner must weigh the costs of staying home versus paying for daycare when you are making this decision. Another option that some couples prefer is for the father to stay home with baby after the first six weeks or so of the mother's maternity leave. This option may be the best for you if her income is significantly higher than yours. If this case describes the situation for you and your partner, your role as stay-at-home dad will be an extremely fulfilling and adventurous experience. There is no substitute for the bond between a father and his child, especially if he is the primary caregiver during the work week.

Above all else, remain sensitive to your partner's emotional needs and be supportive if she suffers from separation anxiety when she returns to work after the birth of your baby. The initial adjustment can be very difficult for her and for your little one. As long as you are ready to be a steady source of emotional calm during this time, your little family will get through this time just fine.

# Packing the Hospital Bags

The conundrum of knowing what to take on vacation and what to leave behind is nothing compared to the quandary of what to take to the hospital when your baby is on her way. Packing the hospital bag is often broken down into three sections – things needed for mom during the birth, things needed for mom after the birth, and things needed for the baby. Things needed for dad often get a bit neglected, because fathers weren't welcome anywhere near the action for a long time. Fortunately, times have changed, and the chances are that you are the best man for the job to get organized about Project Birth. Here are some suggestions for a mom-, baby-, and dad-friendly hospital bag:

# What Parents Need During the Birth

You are going to need some or all of the following items:

- **Camera and batteries:** Make sure you know how to use all the buttons.

- **Cell phone and charger:** Check with the hospital before making phone calls to announce your little one's arrival. Some hospitals do not allow you to use cell phones inside.

- **Music, pictures, and other personal items:** Take anything that you and your partner think will make labor easier by setting a nice mood. Check with your healthcare providers first, because some hospitals may not allow certain personal items in the delivery suite.

- **Snacks and drinks:** Some labors can take a long time (24 hours or more), and it's hard work on mom doing all the pushing and dad doing all that supporting. Nuts, chocolate, energy drinks, power bars, crackers, or whatever you like can be packed in a lunchbox for you to nibble on during the labor. If she's in the hospital, your partner may not be allowed anything more than ice chips, so take your goodies out of her sight when you need to eat or drink.

- **The appropriate clothing:** Mom's feet may get cold during a long labor, so pack a pair of nice, comfortable socks for her. If you're having a water birth, you may want to pack a pair of shorts so you can get in the pool too.

There may be a lot of waiting around, so pack a book or something to keep you occupied. However, remember your primary purpose. Getting into a good book may not be the best way to spend your time when you're supposed to be supporting your partner.

## What Mom Needs After the Birth

In all likelihood, you'll be spending a few hours with your new baby, calling everyone you want to call and feeling a little giddy. You may head home for a shower, something to eat, and some sleep. But mom needs at least these things to help her settle into her stay at the hospital:

- **A comfortable change of clothes** for coming home. It takes some time for a pregnant belly to shrink down enough to fit into pre-pregnancy clothes. Reminding mom of this before she ever leaves the hospital could depress her unnecessarily.

- **Lanolin nipple cream** that doesn't need to be washed off before breastfeeding.

- **Maternity bras and nursing pads** in case of leaking breast milk. For some new moms, milk comes in during the hospital stay. For others, it could take as long as 5 days after the birth for milk to come in so it may not happen until after you have come home with your new baby. Either way, it's best to be prepared.

- **Maternity pads,** although these are often supplied by the hospital.

- **Soft cotton undies**. Maternity underwear may be best, but they should be some that she doesn't mind getting stained. The hospital will probably provide ample pairs of disposable underwear but bring some of her own, so she has the option.

- **A pen and notebook**, in case she would like to record a few things before or after the birth.

- **Pajamas or a nightgown** that opens at the front for breastfeeding, a robe, and slippers. Some women prefer to wear the hospital's gowns at first, so they don't ruin their own clothes with bodily fluids (which are often copious after delivery).

- **Usual toiletries** your partner would take on vacation, such as a toothbrush, shampoo, cleanser, deodorant, moisturizer, lip balm, contact lens supplies, hair bands and brush, and any medications.

# What Baby Needs After Birth

The little person you'll be bringing home will need the following items:

- **Disposable diapers:** Even if you are going to use cloth diapers, meconium, the sticky tarlike stool your baby expels in the first few days after birth, is best handled by disposable diapers. The hospital will probably supply some disposable diapers, but they may be too large or too small, depending on the size of your newborn.

- **Pacifier:** While a pacifier is probably one of the most commonly known baby accessories, lactation consultants may not be happy about you giving your little one a pacifier if you're experiencing breastfeeding difficulties, because pacifiers are believed to cause "nipple confusion" in some cases.

- **Supplies for bottle feeding:** Formula (newborn), bottles, nipples, and a bottle warmer if you're going to bottle feed.

- **Blankets:** It's safer to put a blanket over the baby after he's in his car seat than to put a heavy coat on him. It's difficult to tighten the straps enough to keep him safe if he's wearing heavy outer clothing.

- **Something to wear:** A couple of newborn-sized all-in-ones with feet and long sleeves, some hats, and some socks or booties. Newborns are used to being in a nice hot spa pool and have no way to control their temperature yet, so even in summer, they need to be kept warm. You may also have a special "coming home" outfit picked out.

Check with a lactation consultant for any breastfeeding equipment, aids, or remedies your partner may need.

# Preparing to Support Her During Labor

We've talked a lot about supporting and being there for your partner. So, what does "being there" really mean? Ask a lot of dads who have been through the birth of their children, and the first answer that may spring to mind is "stand around like an idiot and feel guilty and inadequate." It's easy to feel sidelined when the focus is on your partner, and she's in kind of a crabby mood with you, which you would be too if you had seven pounds of a person coming out of an orifice. She's focusing on what her body is doing; listening to the coaching and advice of her midwife, nurses, or obstetrician; and coping with pain, hormones, and emotions, you can't even begin to imagine (and don't want to).

In general, your partner relies on you to sort out a long list of support tasks that you can do with dignity and humility. So, if your partner needs a shoulder to hang on to for leverage when she's pushing, give it to her. If she needs three ice chips and a back rub, get them for her. If she says she can't do it anymore, tell her with conviction that she can. Being there means taking care of your partner when she needs you to, and most importantly, taking charge when she needs you to.

Labor can be totally overwhelming for a woman, and she's vulnerable to every emotion in the book. She's also vulnerable to being pushed around by the hospital system: an obstetrician who may be angling for a cesarean birth when your partner is dead set against it and wants to keep pushing for a bit longer or an overly pushy lactation consultant who is stressing out your exhausted partner. If something doesn't feel right, you have to make a decision for the good of your partner and baby and advocate on their behalf. It's all about your family, so you get to be the man who calls the shots when push comes to shoves.

Dads can really make their role count during labor by being:

- **A link to the outside world:** Let friends and family know what's going on because they will be eager to hear how the birth is going. You can also be the first to announce to the world that your new son or daughter has arrived – a very special role indeed!

- **Strong:** Help out where you can by making sure your partner is as comfortable as she can be, is well-stocked with whatever she needs, and is cool or warm enough.

- **The rational, calm voice in the hustle and bustle:** Even when things get stressful or hectic, try to keep your cool on your partner's behalf and advocate for her if things are slipping out of control.

Take your cues from your partner. Her needs are pretty specific, and she'll let you know about them. But don't try to tell your partner you know how she feels, because you don't. Any complaining (to her) of any sort from your end may not be received well.

You might also want to be ready to have a standby support person in case labor goes on for a long time, or you desperately need some rest. Talk about who would be suitable for your partner. Perhaps her sister or mother could fill in for you while you have a meal or take a breather. You'll be of very little use if you pass out from exhaustion or starvation!

# Assembling Home Birthing Equipment

If you have a hospital birth, you don't need to bring anything other than your partner and your hospital bags. But if you have the birth at home, you need some equipment to prepare for the big day. Your midwife will undoubtedly give you a comprehensive and somewhat daunting list that may include the following items:

- **A birthing pool:** These can be rented or purchased from private companies; your midwife will probably know of a source. Some can even be used as a paddling pool for your child afterward.

- **A container for the placenta,** unless you're planning to bury it in the backyard.

- **Towels:** These are for cleaning up and wrapping the baby in after birth, and for mom and dad if you've both been in the pool.

- **Waterproof mats to cover your carpet:** A tarp covered with newspaper and an old blanket or sheets should do it.

If you can take charge of finding and preparing everything on the list for a home birth, your partner will be more calm, cool, and collected as she gets ready for the big day. The more stress you can take off her shoulders, the better she will feel!

# Last-Minute Preparations

As you approach the final days before your partner's due date, you can be feeling all sorts of things – excitement about meeting your baby for the first time, or absolute terror about the reality of your new responsibility. You may also be a bit worried about how you'll handle the labor, your role in it, and how well your partner will cope. Worrying is okay, and yes, lots of guys cry, pass out, or throw up during labor, which is all part of the journey.

Before the fun starts, double-check a few things, such as ensuring that you've:

- Arranged for someone to look after your pets or plants and bring in your mail (you may be gone for a few days).
- Briefed people at work, or left handover noes or contact details in case you need to leave suddenly.
- Charged your camera batteries or packed charging cords.
- Got the hospital bags packed and ready to go, even if you're planning a home birth, in case you need to transfer to a hospital in a hurry.
- Made sure the car seat is ready to go and have practiced putting it in and taking it out of the car.

- Stored cell phone numbers of friends and family on your cell phone and packed your charger. You should also have emergency numbers on-hand if you need to get in touch with the hospital or your healthcare provider before you head in for delivery.
- Have all the equipment you need at home if you are planning a home birth.
- Ensured that the nursery has the essentials, meaning baby has somewhere to sleep, bedding, clothing, diapers and diaper cream, diaper wipes, and a place for changing diapers.
- Made sure your care has all its paperwork and gas, you know your way to the hospital or birthing center, you have parking money, and you know where parking is. Also, make sure you have a backup person to call for transportation if your car should suddenly be out of commission.

Although nothing can fully prepare you and your partner for the real experience of labor, remember that it is your job to think ahead and plan for as many eventualities as possible. The more prepared and calm you are, the less stressed and overwhelmed your partner will be feeling as the big day approaches. If she's as relaxed and happy as possible, she and your baby will be in better health and have a better chance of experiencing a smooth and healthy delivery.

# Chapter 7: If You're Expecting Multiples

So, you've just found out, through the magic of an ultrasound scan, that you're going to be a father of not one, but two (or more) babies at once. You're freaking out. But you should know that being a dad to two or more at the same time, while it is hard work, is not impossible or completely unmanageable. Think of this opportunity as an excellent chance to be twice the man (at least) that you are today!

## The Miracle of Multiple Births

Having twins, triplets, or more babies at once is called a multiple birth. Multiple births happen in two ways. Identical or monozygotic twins are formed when the fertilized egg divides into two very early on, and two separate embryos develop. Non-identical twins, also known as fraternal or dizygotic twins, occur when two eggs are fertilized at once in the fallopian tubes. Triplets can sometimes be a combination with two identical twins and a fraternal twin, but not always. Two or more fraternal siblings can also sometimes develop simultaneously as a result of in-vitro fertilization, in which multiple embryos can be inserted into the uterus in the hopes that at least one of them will implant and lead to a viable pregnancy.

## Risk Factors Involved with Multiple Births

In pregnancy, twins and other multiple births are at risk of arriving prematurely (38 weeks is considered full term for twins) and having a low birth weight. Your healthcare provider will guide you through the intricacies of multiple births and will probably monitor your partner's well-being throughout the pregnancy much more closely than if she were expecting one baby.

Unfortunately, expecting more than one baby often means that the side effects of being pregnant are more pronounced; morning sickness may be more intense, faster and earlier weight gain in the pregnancy, and things like varicose veins, heartburn, and shortness of breath also getting more noticeable.

Since multiple babies are at risk of preterm birth, you must also be prepared for the possibility of other complications. Babies that are born before they have reached the 37-week mark can have an increased risk of many health problems, both long-term and short-term. Some of the short-term problems can include difficulty with body temperature regulation and problems with breathing and eating. Other potential issues, like behavior disabilities and learning difficulties, will not be apparent until later in the children's lives.

## Precautions Taken with Multiple Pregnancies

Because of the risk of preterm birth, your healthcare provider may prescribe bed rest for your partner towards the end of the pregnancy. Some women must be hospitalized and carefully monitored as their final weeks of pregnancy approach, while others can follow a modified bedrest plan. Adhering to the doctor's recommendations, whether strict bedrest or limiting physical activity, your partner can help prevent preterm labor. Reducing stress and strain can go a long way towards increasing blood flow to the uterus and relieving pressure from the cervix, thus helping to prevent early contractions. While bed rest is typically prescribed later in multiple pregnancies, some women are at such high risk of preterm labor that they must limit their activity starting in the early second trimester.

Many women have an extremely difficult time being confined to a bed, especially if they are typically very active or feel they have a lot to do around the house. That's where you come in, dads. If your partner must rest in bed all day or part of each day, it is critical that you pitch in even more than you already have been. The task of ensuring that your partner remains a serene and relaxed incubator for your precious babies is largely up to you.

Additionally, most doctors recommend that women expecting multiples limit any sexual activity, so they don't accidentally induce preterm labor. For this reason and financial reasons, bedrest can put a damper on your relationship. Any advance preparation you can do, in terms of setting aside money for when she has to be off her feet, gathering supplies, so she is comfortable, and shopping for baby needs as early as possible, will help her feel more at ease once she is confined to bed.

## Finding Support

It will be an excellent idea to seek emotional support if you are expecting multiples. Support groups can help you considerably because other members will have experienced what you are going through. Seasoned parents of multiples can help you know what to expect, how to handle various situations, and be there to provide moral support should any crises arise. You might be able to find a local Multiples of

America club in your area, or you can also seek help from family, friends, churches, and support agencies.

## Enlisting Extra Help

Face it – as a man, you may be very reluctant to ask *anyone* for help. But if you and your partner are expecting more than one baby, you're going to have to set aside your pride and ask a lot of people for help, for the good of your own sanity, your partner's emotional and physical health, and the wellbeing of your coming babies.

Expecting more than one baby means that you'll need to buy two or more sets of almost every baby supply item. Doubling (or tripling) the shopping list is a huge financial burden unless you just happen to be financially independent. Instead of going into debt over cribs and diapers, why not ask for help? You may be surprised at how many people are willing to donate hand-me-downs, help you look for used supplies for sale, buy some diapers, or even organize a baby shower for you and your partner. You're going to have to grow accustomed to saying "thank you" a lot, graciously accepting help, and understanding that you and your partner may not be able to do this all by yourselves. If it takes a village to raise a child, it must take a city to raise twins or triplets!

On top of needing help with supplies, you will likely need a lot of extra hands on deck during the first several weeks after the babies' birth. Since your partner will likely be convalescing from a difficult birth and you may have to return to work, start asking around to find out which friends and family members will be able to help care for the babies. Even though you don't know the exact date of the babies' birth or when you'll get to bring them home from the hospital, you can even start making a tentative schedule of helpers now. For example, you might find out who can help with the babies on different days of the week and during different times of the day. Gather phone numbers and be ready to start calling the people you have lined up when you get a better idea of when you'll need their help. These people can change diapers, help soothe the babies, bring them to your partner for breastfeeding and bonding time, do laundry, make meals for you, help care for the house and any pets, and provide emotional support when you and your partner both feel like walking zombies from sleep deprivation.

Above all, try to continue to be a rock of support for your partner, even though you may be feeling overwhelmed and anxious. You don't need to hide your feelings; by all means, discuss how you're feeling with her. But by proactively making as many preparations as possible and finding lots of support for the two of you, you'll be able to help ease your own fears and help her to feel calmer and more confident as she approaches the birth of your babies.

# Chapter 8: The Big Showdown – It's Go Time

The nursery is ready, the freezer is stocked with meals, the car seat is installed, and you may be pacing around the house waiting for it all to start happening. It's like sitting in a reception room, waiting for your name to be called so you can finally become a dad. Keep yourself occupied with some last-minute tasks and a bit of brushing up on what happens during and immediately after labor.

## The Basics of Labor

You cannot be too prepared for the time when your partner goes into labor. And as you're the number one in the pit crew, understanding what's going on is essential. To help you begin to comprehend this momentous occasion, here's a quick guide to what generally happens during labor. Like pregnancy, labor happens in three stages:

- The **first stage** is when your partner's cervix softens, then widens, called dilation, making space for the baby to come through and out of the uterus. The uterus contracts at regular intervals, allowing the baby to come through. The contractions become increasingly painful. These are the contractions you've heard so much about on TV. The cervix is fully dilated at ten centimeters. For a first birth, the first stage takes an average of 6 to 14 hours (but can take a day or more), so you can see that your presence with a strong shoulder and heat packs or ice packs galore will really help.

- The **second stage** is the pushing stage, and it ends when the baby actually comes out. This process is also helped along by contractions that increase in length and intensity. Finally, your little one is born!

- The **third stage** is a little less glamorous and involves the placenta, that lifeline of your baby, being delivered. The placenta is also called afterbirth. It takes from five minutes to an hour to appear after the baby does. Most women are too exhausted by this stage or energized by finally meeting their baby, to notice much about expelling the placenta.

Think that's all there is to it? Nope! The first stage also has three phases, and your partner will probably be too caught up in the moment to recognize them as they happen to her:

- **Latent phase:** Contractions are 5 to 20 minutes apart and become more frequent as they progress. The cervix dilates to about 3 centimeters.

- **Active phase:** This phase is characterized by the cervix dilating from about 3 centimeters to fully dilated. Contractions increase in length and intensity, coming every three to five minutes and lasting about 60 seconds, so your partner doesn't have a lot of down time to think about anything. It's up to you to recognize what's happening and get things organized. This is usually when getting to the hospital or opening the door for the midwife to deliver your baby at home is right up there on your to-do list.

- **Transition:** Okay, your partner is allowed to lose it now – and probably will. This is the point just before the pushing starts. Contractions are very intense, sometimes overwhelming, and your partner may say some unpleasant or downright insulting things, including some aimed directly at you. Don't worry – this too shall pass!

One of the most obvious signs that things are about to kick off is when your partner's water breaks. This can happen in an inappropriate situation, but it happens to a lot of pregnant women, so don't be too embarrassed when the big box store you're browsing has to call for a "cleanup on aisle one." However, labor does not always follow immediately on the heels of membrane rupture. It may, but in some cases, labor starts up to 24 hours after her water breaks. Either way, call your doctor or midwife to inform them that her water has broken; in some cases, your doctor may want her to come to the hospital to be checked.

## Helping to Time the Contractions

In some cases, your healthcare provider will want you to monitor your partner's contractions until they follow the 5-1-1 rule – that is, they are five minutes apart, lasting for one minute each, and they have been that way for one hour. At this point, they will want you to come into the hospital or birthing center, preferably calling to notify them ahead of time that you are on the way.

Sometimes you'll go through a few false alarms before labor is really progressing, meaning that your partner will have episodes of Braxton-Hicks contractions. These contractions, while very real and sometimes painful, are typically irregular and eventually fade in intensity over time. You can think of them as "practice" contractions as the uterus gets ready for the real event. They can occur anytime in the second half of the pregnancy or even earlier, but often women experience them frequently in the days and weeks leading up to labor.

Whether she is experiencing the contractions of early labor or Braxton-Hicks contractions, you will need to help monitor their timing to help determine if you need to go to the hospital. It should not surprise you that there are cell phone apps specifically designed to help you monitor the duration and frequency of your partner's contractions. If you do a search on your phone's app store, you should find plenty of options. Investigate a few of them long before the big day so you can decide which one you like best. Then, when your partner begins to feel the signs of early labor, you can open the app and start timing! She'll really appreciate your insight and preparedness.

# When You Think It's Really Starting

Before your partner's water breaks and true contractions begin, you will have signs that the birth of your baby is not far away, but it can still be days or weeks before full-on labor really starts. At this point in the pregnancy, you and your partner are likely feeling quite impatient to meet your little one. No matter how tired and frustrated you are from the preparations and waiting; you need to understand that your partner is probably a hundred times more uncomfortable and readier for the pregnancy to be over. If you see the following signs, you can take them as a good sign of things progressing and give her some encouragement. Remind her of how strong she is and that there is just a little more time before she will get to hold your precious baby in her arms. She'll be impressed and grateful that you took the time to learn the signs and symptoms of impending labor, even though some of them are a bit disgusting. Here's what to look for:

- **A bloody show or mucus plug:** The mucus plug that blocks the cervix during pregnancy comes away, along with blood from broken capillaries in the cervix. This usually happens when the cervix starts to dilate slightly and can occur weeks before labor actually starts, especially if this is your partner's first pregnancy.

- **Braxton-Hicks contractions:** See the previous description.

- **Intense or increasing back pain:** This pain can be a sign that things are beginning to happen. Some women actually experience all or most of the pain and discomfort of contractions in their backs.

- **Loose bowel movements:** A few days before labor, the body releases prostaglandins, which help soften the cervix in preparation for dilation. They also can cause things to be a bit lax in the bowel department.

Don't worry if none of the things in the preceding list happens before your partner's contractions start. Each labor, birth, and woman is different, and some symptoms are felt so subtly at first that they are not even noticed. Call your care provider if you are uncertain about what is happening.

When the first stage of labor begins, it may feel like birth is really happening, but it isn't yet. The difference between the latent phase (also sometimes called early labor) and the active phase (sometimes called active labor) of the first stage of labor is the length and intensity of contractions. Call your midwife, obstetrician, or other caregivers for support. She can give you guidance on whether you need to grab the car keys, settle in for the evening, or stay on full alert with a stopwatch (or your phone) in your hand.

# When Things Really Get Going

All aboard the roller coaster need to get buckled in because you are in for a real treat now. The birth of a child happens everywhere around the world thousands of times a day. But you can bet that every birth story happening at each moment is unique. Lucky you, you get to be a part of your baby's story right now! You'll be able to tell him the story for years to come as you celebrate his birthday. The high of seeing a child born is like nothing on Earth – and you are about to meet your own child. How cool is that??

First things first, you'll know your partner is in labor because:

- Contractions are regular, lasting 45 to 60 seconds and increasing in frequency.
- Contractions are getting stronger, and your partner may not be able to speak during a contraction.
- Progressive cervical dilation (usually measured by your healthcare provider) is occurring.

# Helping Her Cope with the Pain

Many women spend the latent phase of labor at home when they're more comfortable and have a lot of room to move around. Even if you're planning a hospital birth, it may pay to stay at home for as long as is feasible. Some women who go to the hospital too early tense up because they're at the hospital and later on experience fatigue earlier than if they'd stayed at home in longer. Studies have shown that women who spend more time at home during the latent phase of labor (see the previously stated 5-1-1 rule for when to go into the hospital) tend to have easier labor experiences overall, generally with fewer medical interventions. Having said that, some women who have experienced a difficult pregnancy or are at risk for birth complications will be asked to come into the hospital at the slightest indication of labor. Make sure you are aware of and understand the specific recommendations for your partner before the big day is here.

Whether you're having the birth at home or in a hospital, you may be able to try some or all of these techniques to help your partner manage the pain naturally during labor. If you are unsure about any of them, check with your healthcare provider first:

- Apply a hot water bottle to your partner's lower back or wherever she feels the most pain.
- Give your partner a gentle back rub with some almond or olive oil. She may even prefer that you put some moderate to firm pressure against her hips or lower back during contractions; ask her if she would like for you to try this technique.
- Help her sit up in place – while holding very still – if she decides to have epidural anesthesia. Encourage her and remind her of how strong she is, because holding completely still while experiencing stabbing pain is no small feat!
- Keep your partner moving, if she's up to it. If you're home, try walking slowly around the block a few times with her. If you're in the hospital, she may be able to pace the hallway with you. Movement can help labor progress, and gravity helps the baby's weight put pressure on the cervix, helping it to dilate.
- Run a bath or offer to turn on the shower for your partner. If her water has broken, her care provider may not want her to get into the tub, so ask first.
- Dim the lights and try playing some music or soothing sounds of her choice. Try to prepare in advance by asking her what kind of music she may appreciate

during labor. Of course, once labor has started, she may change her mind about what helps and what doesn't!

As contractions get stronger and you move into the active phase, transition, and the second stage of labor, these pain-relief techniques can greatly help you carry on with the pregnancy. Let your partner guide you as to what she needs. At some points, she won't have any energy in her body to do anything other than ride out the contraction, especially in the second stage when she's putting everything into pushing the baby out. Holding your partner's body and letting her lean on you in whatever way she needs to may help her a lot. In other words, be an active, not passive, participant of the labor process.

## Keeping Your Sanity – and Hers

Labor can take a long time. You may get a chance to have a breather between contractions, or you may not. Giving all your energy to your partner is exhausting, so try to take some time out for yourself if you can. Taking quick breathers will help ensure that you remain strong, engaged, and encouraging for her.

It may help to have a couple people on speed-dial that you can call if it all becomes too much.

Check with your partner before the big day, because it would be terrible to have a person turn up during labor which your partner really doesn't want to see there.

Acceptable and/or recommended things for dads to do during labor include:

- Supporting your partner's decisions – to take pain medication or not, to have an epidural or not. Even if some of these decisions may not have been on your partner's original birth plan, remain open and flexible so you can support her no matter what she needs. Before labor, it's hard for a woman to predict her own pain tolerance and what will or will not be helpful at the moment.

- Crying when the baby is here.
- Doing some stretching exercises to keep fresh and fend off sleep.
- Drinking water.
- Eating snacks (not in front of your partner, unless she's allowed to eat too).
- Fainting (warn the nurses first so they can move all equipment out of the way).
- Getting some fresh air – as long as it's brief.
- Going to the toilet (if it's not too often and doesn't take too long).

- Leaving the room if you're about to be sick or faint.
- Advocating for her desires and decisions if you feel the healthcare staff are not listening to her. Sometimes they have to act quickly and in opposition to her desires for the sake of her health or the health of your baby, so remember to be open-minded and reasonable.
- Acting as a "body-guard" and politely refusing to allow well-meaning friends and family members access to the room unless they are people you and your partner have invited in advance to be a part of the labor process. Everyone else can wait until the baby is born and your partner is ready to start introducing him to the rest of the world.

## Medical Interventions

Sometimes during labor nature needs a helping hand to get your baby out into the world. There are lots of reasons for this. The baby may be in distress, or your partner's health is in jeopardy, or she's exhausted and wants the baby out immediately. None of these interventions can really be anticipated. Keep in touch with your partner, and if she's adamant that she doesn't want any intervention, help be her advocate. When the medical equipment comes out, try not to freak out. Some of it can look scarier than it really is. The equipment's going to help you meet your baby sooner rather than later.

The following interventions may be necessary for helping the process along:

- **Induction:** If your partner is past her due date with no signs of impending labor, or if your healthcare provider believes delivery should not be delayed due to any health concerns for mother or baby, she may be placed on an IV drip of a hormone called Pitocin. This substance mimics the natural hormone oxytocin to get the process of labor started.

- **Manually breaking the amniotic sac:** If labor has progressed to a certain point and then stalled, the doctor may carefully rupture the amniotic sac (causing your partner's water to break) to help get things going.

- **Vacuum extraction:** A vacuum extractor helps pull the baby out of the birth canal if the baby's head is low in the birth canal but needs an extra bit of oomph to help him along. The baby's heart rate may indicate he's in distress, or his position is making it tricky for him to be born naturally. A suction cup is placed on the baby's head, and your partner may have to have an episiotomy, which is a cut to the vaginal opening to make room for the cup to go in. This type of delivery can cause swelling to the top of the baby's head, but usually causes little or no trauma to mother and baby.

- **Forceps:** These look like a scary pair of tongs. They are used to grip the baby's head on both sides and pull him out of the birth canal. These aren't used as often as the vacuum these days because of the risk that the mother's insides can be damaged, not to mention the bruising and risk of damage to the baby's head. An episiotomy is usually required as well.

- **Emergency cesarean:** A surgical delivery is the ultimate medical intervention. It's called "emergency" to distinguish it from elective cesareans, which are scheduled in advance. All cesareans take place in an operating room, so you'll have to dress for the part by wearing a gown and covering your face and hair. Your partner is given an epidural or spinal anesthetic to numb pain (although in some cases general anesthetic is necessary), and an incision is made in your partner's belly, usually near the pubic bone. The abdominal muscles are parted, and the peritoneal cavity is opened to make way for the uterus. The uterus is then opened, and the baby and placenta are brought out.

Having a cesarean is not an easy way of having a baby; it's major surgery, and it also means that your partner will endure a longer recovery than if she was able to give birth vaginally. She will not be able to drive or lift anything heavy for up to six weeks. She will also be on pain medications and will need to rest a lot as she recovers. Her hospital stay is also likely to be a bit longer.

If your partner had her heart set on a vaginal birth or a natural, drug-free birth and it hasn't worked out that way, she may be feeling disappointed and upset with herself. Add this to the hormones rampaging through her body, and you may have one super emotional new mama. Give her all the love and support you can muster, because she needs you now. Remind her that she did an amazing job, no matter how the birth went, and the important part is that she and your precious little one finally get to see each other for the first time.

## The Big Moment

The moment your child is born is difficult to describe – totally unique, beautiful, and out of this world. Enjoy it fully. You may find that you shed a tear or two at this important moment. If this is the case, don't hold back or be embarrassed. Remember to snap a few quick pictures of the moment your child is handed to your partner or placed on her chest. She will also cherish a picture of when your new baby is weighed and measured.

## Cutting the Cord

This part of the process is your brief moment to be in the spotlight. You have an important job to do, should you choose to accept it, and if your care provider offers (sometimes complications make this part unadvisable). After the baby is born, then the doctor will clamp the cord and set it up for you to cut. This part symbolizes the end of pregnancy and the start of your partner's new role as this baby's mother. For you, it may represent your part in your new family.

The cord is somewhat thick and gnarly, so apply a little elbow grease and give it a good strong cut. You may want to ask one of the healthcare staff members to take a quick photo.

Your caregiver may need to suction fluid from your baby's mouth or nose, or massage her back with a warm cloth, to help her breath. Within the first few minutes after birth, an Apgar test will be done on her. This test gives babies scores on five basic criteria and alerts care providers to any concerns about the baby's health. Finally, your caregiver dries your baby and (hopefully) hands her over to mom for some skin-on-skin bonding time. Sometimes this is not possible due to health concerns, but most hospitals follow this practice because it is best for both mother and baby.

## The First Few Hours

After weighing and measuring your baby, giving matching identification bracelets to mother and baby, and taking a quick footprint from the baby, many healthcare providers will give your little family some alone time at this point, as long as there are no pressing health concerns. At some point before or after mom cuddles with the baby, you'll get a chance to meet and hold your little one for the first time. It can be amazing, scary, bewildering, and incomprehensible all at once. Take a moment to appreciate your beautiful new addition to the family and marvel at his tiny features. Mom may be busy being taken care of the medical staff right now, so cherish your first minutes of bonding with your new child. Typically, there is no rush anymore once your baby has been checked and is handed to you, so take some time to make your first acquaintance with the little one.

## Practical Matters

Once all the commotion has died down, there are a few practical matters to attend to. Have you started calling friends and family yet? Mom and baby usually spend an hour or more cuddling, getting to know each other, and having something to eat. Feeding your baby is going to be mom's number one priority for some time now, so they need to get into it right away. Sometimes a care provider will help mom and baby get comfy with a first breastfeed or helps with the mechanics of getting your baby to take a bottle if you've decided to formula feed.

Next on the agenda are usually the tasks of getting baby dressed and helping mom into clean, comfortable clothes. Nurses are often on hand to help her to the bathroom to get cleaned up. Later, you may need to give her a hand standing up and getting around, especially if she's had an epidural during labor.

A bit of food and drink for mom is usually in order now, too. It may have been a long time since either of you had a decent meal. Taking care of any food cravings your partner couldn't eat during labor may be high on your agenda. Finally, all the two of you may feel like now is some well-deserved rest. Try to see to it that any hospital formalities are dealt with quickly so your new little family can get some rest. Enjoy a few hours of quiet, if possible – you have all worked extremely hard, and you deserve it!

## The First Few Days

Many parents have been lulled into thinking their baby is a perfect angel in the first 24 hours. Babies can be very sleepy and settled for the first day, and you may be fooled! But it's also a very busy time getting feeding patterns established and finding your feet in your new role as a dad. Your baby should have at least six feedings in a 24-hour period to start with (this will increase), so supporting mom by taking care of diaper changes, burping, or anything else that needs attending to can help her out a lot. If mom is still in the hospital, you can be a real hero by spending a lot of extra time with the baby, so your partner can rest some more. Many hospitals allow dads to room-in with mother and baby.

## Going Home

If your baby was born in a hospital, your care provider and the hospital decide when your partner and baby can go home. For some new moms, going home can't come fast enough. For others, additional time in the hospital may help her recover adequately from the birth and prepare for the task of caring for the baby. Don't let the hospital push you out if you're not ready for it. Talk about your concerns with your caregiver, but keep in mind that you can't stay in the relative safety of the hospital forever!

# Chapter 9: What to Expect the First Few Weeks

Your baby is finally here. Does being a dad feel real now? If not, don't worry. The first few days and weeks after birth can feel surreal. It does get better, though. If you felt a bit left out during pregnancy and birth, now is your time to show your worth and help out as much as possible. Your baby needs lots of bonding time with his dad!

## Caring for Baby and Helping Your Partner

Every baby is different, and every family is different. In the coming days, weeks, and months, you'll discover how to read and care for your child like no one else ever will – except for Mom, that is. Now is the time to put into practice all the training you received for caring for your baby. Much of it will be trial and error. Don't worry; there is no such thing as a perfect parent. Everyone has made plenty of silly parenting mistakes, especially in the early days, and their children have survived and thrived despite these errors.

The most vital thing you can do is help your partner as much as possible. She is going to be exhausted and hormonal from the experience of the birth for several days or even weeks, especially if she had a cesarean delivery. As a result, you'll still need to do the lion's share of household work without complaint. It will take quite a bit of time before she is able to be up and about to her pre-pregnancy abilities.

If you are bottle feeding, you can share equally in feeding your baby, especially at night. Taking turns with feeding is one of the best ways to help the two of you cope with the unbelievable strain of sleep deprivation you'll experience in the first several weeks of parenthood. If your partner is breastfeeding, you can still help tremendously by changing the diaper and making sure baby is clean and dressed before handing him off to mom for a feeding.

Other ways in which you can help are making sure mom and baby get to scheduled check-ups, cooking meals, and making sure any well-meaning guests don't overstay their welcome. Everyone will be eager to meet your new little one, but your priority should be making sure your partner does not get overwhelmed, and the baby is not disturbed or overstressed by too many guests. Try to space out visitors, so you don't see more than one or two people each day, and set aside certain days in which you receive no visitors, so your new family can bond and relax together.

# Baby Blues or Something More Serious?

About day three after birth, mom may start feeling a bit low. This is perfectly normal and should pass. She may burst into tears for no reason that she can explain or just feel overwhelmed by responsibility. If she had a hard pregnancy and is looking forward to getting her body back, finding it isn't "back" yet may be very disappointing. Chances are she will also be sore in all sorts of places. Performing simple personal hygiene tasks or even just going to the toilet can be really tricky and uncomfortable. On top of all that is the fact that her hormone levels have gone through yet another dramatic shift, which significantly affects her mood and body. Do your dad thing and try to support your partner by helping out, telling her she's amazing and enjoying your baby.

These initial baby blues have nothing to do with postpartum depression, which is likely to come later if your partner ends up experiencing it. Feeling "the blues" is one thing, being in a black hole is another. That's how some people describe postpartum depression (PPD). The condition is associated with mothers for the most part, with an estimated 10 to 15 percent of mothers suffering from PPD. What's less well-known is that three to ten percent of fathers can suffer from PPD, too. This is a serious condition that cannot be ignored without significant consequences.

## Recognize the Signs of PPD

Knowing about and recognizing some of the signs of PPD can assist you to seek help for yourself or your partner if either of you experience PPD. Symptoms to look for include the following:

- Anxiety or panic attacks.
- Feelings of hopelessness.
- Frequent crying spells.
- Loss of energy or appetite.
- Loss of enjoyment in everyday activities or your baby.
- Loss of sex drive.
- Mood swings.
- The trouble with sleeping even when the baby is settled.
- Prolonged feelings of sadness, with nothing to look forward to.
- Suicidal thoughts.

Every case is different. If you feel you or your partner may have PPD, talk to each other about how you're feeling and see your doctor.

# Getting Help

If your partner has PPD, supporting her may seem like an impossible task, but you can help in lots of ways. Try some of these ideas:

- Arrange a time for you to spend together, just the two of you. Regular "us" time can help destress both of you and share some common ground again.
- Let her talk while you listen, or involve a friend she feels comfortable talking to.
- Take over more of the housework and baby care so she can try to get some sleep. If you can't take on everything, enlist the support of family and friends.
- Treat her to a special gift, a date night, or some pampering at a spa.
- Make sure she is following up with any therapies, doctor appointments, or medications needed.

For additional PPD support and help for either one of you, try some of the following ideas:

- Talk to your doctor. He can offer a wide range of options like counseling or medications. He may also know of local sources for support groups.
- Find support in your community — many hospitals host groups dealing with PPD. Online groups can also be a lifesaver.

- Get some exercise. Feeling fit and active can lift your mood or the mood of your partner. Around 30 minutes of daily activity is all that is needed to release mood-enhancing hormones.
- Talk to family and friends. You might be amazed at how anxious people are to help, and many of them may have had similar experiences.

Postpartum depression is temporary, and you can find a way to help yourself or your partner through it. If you feel lost, take stock and get some help.

## Keep Communicating!

Make sure you and your partner communicate well, no matter how stressful things get. Touch bases frequently to be sure you are on the same page regarding feeding the baby, changing diapers, and beginning to establish a routine. Find out how she's feeling about returning to work, if that was her plan, and be supportive if she needs to voice her unsteady emotions. More than anything else, keeping the communication lines open will help you and your partner remain close and work as a team as you navigate the unknown waters of new parenthood together.

# Conclusion

Thank you for making it through to the end of *"Pregnancy: Put Yourself in Her Shoes."* Let's hope that it was informative and able to provide you with all the tools you need to achieve your goals of being the most supportive partner and new father possible.

The next step is to keep learning how to be an amazing dad and partner throughout your child's life. Every day will bring new learning and growth opportunities. Now that you are a father, life will never dull again. You are in for the adventure of a lifetime! Since you have already proven yourself to be interested in being the rock-solid support to your partner throughout pregnancy, labor, and delivery, you are likely to be a highly successful and supportive father. No matter what life throws at your family, you have shown that you are willing to educate yourself, be sympathetic to the needs of your partner and child, and provide for their needs above all else. Men like you are an inspiration for fathers and fathers-to-be everywhere. If only more partners took the initiative that you have shown, women everywhere would be experiencing happier, healthier, and less stressful pregnancies.

If you have found the information in this book to be beneficial for your own experience, pass it on to friends and family members who are also expecting their first children. Their partners will thank you for helping them learn how to walk a mile in their shoes and better understand the ins and outs of pregnancy.

Finally, if you found this book useful in any way, a review on Amazon is always appreciated!

# Description

Have you just discovered that you're going to be a dad for the first time, and you don't know what to do first? You're not alone! Many first-, second-, or third-time fathers have found themselves wondering what goes on inside their pregnant partner's body, what causes those crazy cravings and emotions, and whether labor really hurts that bad (hint: yes, it does hurt *that bad!*). They find themselves wishing they knew how to be sympathetic to their partners' needs and help them have as smooth of a pregnancy, labor, and delivery as possible. However, they cannot read their partner's minds, and they're not sure how they can be supportive or helpful. If this description sounds like your experience, this eBook is for you!

Inside, you'll discover:
- A summary of pregnancy side effects during each trimester and how you can help ease her discomfort
- How to take an active role in preparing your home for your little one
- Special ways that you can let your partner know that you support and love her unconditionally
- How to be her fiercest advocate throughout the labor and delivery process.

- Helpful checklists for everything – from supplies you need for the baby to what you should bring to the hospital
- How to prepare your mindset for fatherhood
- *And so much more!*